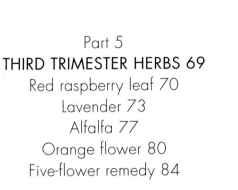

Introduction

In each stage of pregnancy, from the tentative preconception months to the first incredible weeks with your newborn, there are simple, natural ways to ease the stress, counter some of the symptoms and generally boost well-being. Their ingredients couldn't be easier to use and your kitchen cupboards and windowboxes may already be stocked with them.

Herbs have an incredibly long and important history in medicine. They have been used since ancient times to disinfect wounds, boost the immune system and for their tonic effects – and they are still widely employed today. Trials have proven just how effective, for example, ginger can be for easing pregnancy sickness and the power of garlic in boosting immunity.

As in all herbals since the times of the great British herbalists, John Gerard and Nicholas Culpeper in the 16th and 17th centuries, the term 'herb' is extremely broad. It encompasses everything from tree products such as lemons and apples, to roots like dandelion and garlic, pollen by-products such as honey and marine plants like seaweed.

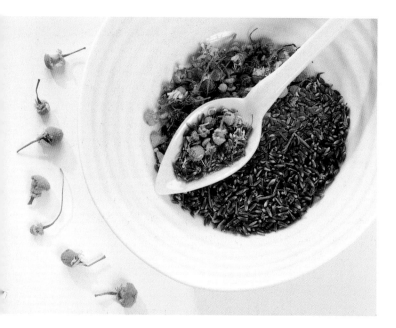

In this book, I have used the broadest definition of the term 'herb' to mean any species of plant that has therapeutic properties.

Herb profiles

Within the chapters of this book, you will find many delicious, soothing and restorative ways to use herbs as well as recommended homeopathic remedies and flower essences, which are all safe to take in pregnancy and without adverse side effects.

Not only are these natural substances helpful during the traditional three trimesters of pregnancy but also in the time leading up to conception, during your postnatal period and throughout the early weeks of your baby's life. You will find, for example, rose-scented massage oil to encourage libido in the preconception weeks, seaweed soaks to boost energy levels as your belly grows, and jasmine treatments to increase your feelings of confidence and assertiveness in the postnatal period.

Each profiled herb is accompanied by an overview of how it is used in the West to promote and maintain pregnancy and during the postnatal period as well as its importance in alternative systems; including Traditional Chinese Medicine, Indian Ayurveda and Indonesian Jamu. Where appropriate, some of the rich lore connected with pregnancy and childbirth that surrounds many of these plants is also included.

Growing and using herbs

It is possible to raise many herbs at home – some thrive in containers and windowboxes or even as houseplants – so you don't need a garden to benefit from their effects. Indeed, some staples of the pregnancy herb kit like dandelions and nettles grow so freely that they are considered weeds. When you have access to fresh herbs, a healing remedy can be as easy as picking a couple of leaves, and either putting them into a mug and pouring over boiling water or casting them into the bath. You will find guidance here on the best time to pick the herbs you grow and on how to dry and store them for therapeutic use.

Other herbs are much simpler to buy in ready-made preparations; these include honey and flower waters. After all, who wants extra hassle when pregnancy and life with a new baby bring so many new priorities? So the chapters also recommend many off-the-shelf products, including

organic teabags, beautycare preparations, tinctures and massage oil blends.

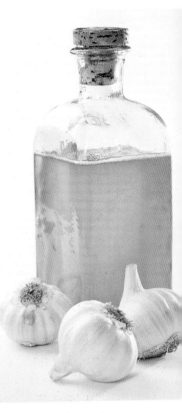

But at the heart of the book are herbal products to be made at home. Nothing is complicated and no specialist equipment is required – just the regular pans, jars and heatproof bowls you already have in your kitchen. It's surprisingly easy, not to say cheap, to make your own beautycare products, for example, particularly at a time when you may want to reduce the number of synthetic chemicals you apply to your skin, or to make your regime organic and sourced from quality ingredients. You will find recipes for healthy foods, too, from salads through to delicious drinks. And there are recipes for all-natural home cleansing products which may appeal to the nesting instinct that can kick in at the most unexpected times in pregnancy.

> **CAUTION** Herbs and essential oils may be natural, but they should be regarded as medicines, with powerful actions, potential side effects and interactions with prescribed or over-the-counter medications. Some are emmenagogues and abortifacients (stimulating menstruation and blood flow in the uterus and pelvis or causing miscarriage) while others may be teratogens (harmful to the healthy development of a baby); others can irritate the skin, or adversely affect body systems or organs. Some are simply toxic.
>
> Where appropriate, specific notes are given with individual herb profiles but, in all cases:
> * Use only the herbs detailed in this book and only as described
> * Use only those parts of the herb outlined here and only in the appropriate trimester
> * Never exceed stated doses of any herb
> * Never take essential oils internally
> * Don't give any herbal drink regularly to a baby under six months; don't give honey to babies under a year old
> * Let your caregiver know you are using herbal products on yourself and your baby
> * If in any doubt about any herbal preparation, seek specialist advice

Herbs and my family

Herbs have always been a part of my life; I use them both at home and in my work writing on natural aspects of pregnancy and babycare.

My daughters, who were raised in a home, stocked with herbs, constantly surprise me with what they've picked up. When they have grazes, they love to smear on our local honey; when they feel under the weather they ask for ginger tea; when they have itchy skin, they smother themselves in olive oil; and for insect bites and rashes, they enjoy snapping aloe vera leaves and extracting the gel. That living heritage is what appeals most to me about the healing powers of herbs.

Susannah Marriott

Part 1

YOUR PREGNANCY HERBAL KIT

Equipment needs, advice on buying and storing herbs, and basic preparation methods for remedies

Basic equipment

Apart from a good pair of secateurs or sharp scissors for harvesting fresh herbs and a trug or basket for transporting them so that they don't get crushed or bruised, most of the equipment you need to make herbal remedies can be found in the kitchen.

Measures

Herbs are usually measured in grams and millilitres; electronic scales that measure as little as 1 g will give the best results. It's also wise to invest in a measuring spoon; in this book 1 tsp equals 5 ml and 1 tbsp equals 3 tsp or 15 ml. A glass pipette marked in millilitres is handy for picking up small quantities of liquids. You will also need a glass measuring jug.

Storage bottles and jars

Dried herbs and prepared remedies should be kept in glass. Unlike plastic, glass is chemically stable and does not leach its ingredients into the preparation stored inside. Avoid metal storage containers, too, which can taint herbs and remedies with a metallic taste. Dark glass is best because it protects its contents from sunlight, which can cause oxidation and affect the efficacy of remedies. You will need jars with airtight lids for storing dried ingredients and cork stoppers for storing some liquids, such as syrups, to allow for the possibility of fermentation (which can cause screw-top lids to explode).

Keeping glass storage jars sterile preserves the lifespan of their contents and helps to prevent fermentation and mould growth. Heat the oven to 170°C/325°F. Wash the jars in hot soapy water, then rinse with boiling water, but do not dry. Using tongs, move the jars to a baking sheet and place in the oven for 10 minutes. Remove using tongs; do not touch the clean jars or they will no longer be sterile.

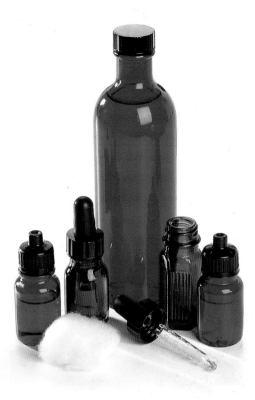

Mixers and strainers

Use glass, stainless steel or enamel bowls, spoons and forks for mixing and stirring. Avoid aluminium utensils, which can taint the finished products. A glass or stoneware pestle and mortar are useful for grinding seeds and making pastes.

A simple fine-meshed plastic sieve is good enough to catch roots, stems and woodier material. For teas and tisanes, a tea strainer works well, but for less mess, use a mesh ball that infuses in the cup. The more delicate green aerial parts of plants will require a finer meshed strainer – it's simplest to place a piece of muslin in a sieve (making sure it is large enough to drape over the rim) and then press flowers and leaves into it using the back of a wooden spoon.

To transfer liquids into storage bottles, you may need a funnel. And if using herbs in the bath, fit a metal strainer over the plug hole to collect debris and prevent blocked drains.

USING A JELLY BAG

A good alternative to a sieve is a jelly bag. You will need to secure the sides around the rim of a glass jar with a thick elastic band or garden twine. Pour in the infusion or decoction and allow plenty of time for the herbal liquid to drip through. Leave plenty of space, too, between the bottom of the bag and base of the jar.

Buying herbs and products

Whether you are buying dried or fresh herbs or tinctures or teas, always buy from a reputable concern — a specialist nursery or herbal or health-food store. Suppliers that sell herbs from dark jars and have a quick turnover or who can recommend (or even have) 'resident' medicinal herbalists and aromatherapists can usually be trusted. When shopping online, first research the ingredient on a site that is not selling any products. Email any questions to the supplier; a reputable firm will always answer your queries.

Buying herbs

Herbs should be bright in colour and have a distinct aroma (and taste). When buying dried herbs, opt for

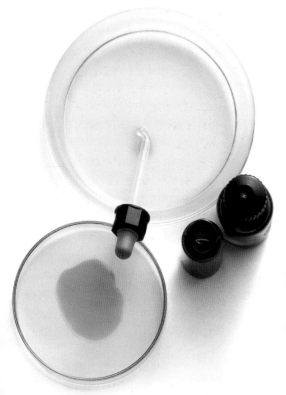

whole leaves and flowers over ground or powdered – they will stay fresher for longer and are less likely to have been adulterated. Check the label for the botanical name and the part of the plant used, for example, the root or leaves, which may have different medicinal actions. If this information is not displayed, the supplier is not treating herbs with the seriousness they demand and it would be better to source ingredients elsewhere.

Herbs raised organically are the most reassuring for use in pregnancy since they are less likely to contain traces of pesticides and heavy metals. Products sporting the logos of the Soil Association and Demeter International comply with strict rules about the use of pesticides and fertilisers. Finally, check the best-before date or date of manufacture.

Botanicals and herbal teas are not scrutinised and tested for safety in the way that over-the-counter and prescription medicines are, nor are they government regulated or standardised like conventional medications. Manufacturers don't have to test or get approval from any official body before bringing them on to the market. As a consequence, herbal ingredients and remedies may be contaminated with heavy metals, pesticides, bacteria or plant matter other than that stated on the label. They may also vary in strength and purity from the claims on the label or website and between batches.

The European Directive on Traditional Herbal Medicinal Products requires that herbal remedies are manufactured to agreed standards of safety and quality that are consistent across Europe. Products new to market need a licence showing that they conform to these agreed standards.

There are no overall regulations governing herbs and remedies originating in the United States, but you can look up selected named brands on the Dietary Supplements Labels Database (see page 125) to verify uses, how the herbs work and adverse effects. You can also check for the latest research trials at the National Center for Complementary and Alternative Medicine (NCCAM) website and the Office of Dietary

Supplements (see page 125). US supplements and botanicals may bear the USP Verified Mark, a sign that remedies have been verified for quality, purity and potency by the United States Pharmacopeia. This non-profit-making volunteer body sets standards that are recognised in 130 countries and ensures that herbal remedies and supplements have consistent chemical markers from batch to batch, meet label claims about strength and purity, and have been manufactured according to good international practices.

Buying herbal remedies

Teas are sold loose or in bags, and may be referred to as infusions or 'tisanes' (an infusion or decoction of any plant other than the common tea plant, *Camellia sinensis*). It's best to choose single herb teas over blends, unless they have been blended by a medicinal herbalist.

A decoction, like a tea, is water-based but is simmered for longer and is likely to have been made from the tougher, woodier parts of the plant, such as the roots or bark.

HERBS TO AVOID

❋ Dusty or mouldy herbs or those lacking an aroma
❋ Herbs containing traces of other matter, such as soil, grass and tiny stones
❋ Herbs stored in clear glass bottles or in direct sunlight

A tincture is a herbal liquid made by steeping the herb in alcohol or an alcohol-and-water solution. It has a longer shelf life than other products (but should be no more than three years old).

Herbs are also sold in tablet and capsule form, known as extracts. It's best to avoid these in pregnancy since the active ingredients can be extremely concentrated.

When buying skincare products made from herbal ingredients, the terms 'organic' and 'herbal' mean nothing without certification from a body like the Soil Association, whose rules govern manufacturing processes, the use of additives, and the quality of the ingredients. In organic products, don't settle for less than 95 per cent organic ingredients.

Buying essential oils

Extracted from flowers and leaves, fruit and berries, bark and resins, essential oils are the highly concentrated essence of a plant, and may have a different action from those parts used by medicinal herbalists. They are extremely potent and must be diluted before use in a base, or carrier, oil. Only use the oils specified and never use more drops than recommended.

When choosing essential oils, it's important to buy those intended for therapeutic use rather than oils distilled for perfumery, soap-making or flavouring, which may use different plant varieties or be synthetically created (and therefore of no medicinal value). The best oils should be marked 'therapeutic grade'; the terms DOP or DEP

HYDROSOLS

A hydrosol is the water left over after the essential oils have been distilled and contains more of the active ingredients than found in flower waters intended for culinary use.

(dipropylene glycol and diethyl phthalate) on the ingredients list are telltale signs of adulteration.

Check the label to make sure you are buying the correct botanical species and that the oil is within its sell-by date. The label may also state the method of extraction, such as steam-distillation or cold-pressed – notes in the individual entries will tell you which one to favour.

Some essential oils, such as rose and neroli, are incredibly expensive but reputable suppliers can often provide ready-blended mixes at different potencies, which makes them affordable. Cheaper options tend to be synthetic or adulterated with cheaper oils. Oils vary in price even from the same supplier – for example, different varieties of lavender from different parts of the world command different price points. Don't trust a supplier who has only one price per oil.

When buying base oils for making massage blends, oil baths and diluting essential oils, think extra-virgin olive oil first. Try to avoid sunflower, soy, corn, safflower, canola and all-purpose 'vegetable' oils.

Making herbal preparations

It's easy and cheap to make your own herbal preparations, but if you find the measuring confusing or the sterilising just too much trouble during pregnancy or when you have a small baby, don't feel guilty. You can always buy ready-made remedies from a reputable herbal supplier.

AN INFUSION

An infusion is the simplest form of herbal preparation – just pour boiling water over fresh or dried leaves, flowers or small seeds. Sip as a tea – either hot or cold, use as a wash or bath for the skin or hair, or soak a cloth in it and use to sponge the skin or as a compress on tired or aching parts.

Always use boiling water when making an infusion, to kill any bacteria in the plant. Herbal teas don't usually need milk, but do add a little honey if you prefer a sweet brew. For those infusions that need long steeping, perhaps even overnight, use a jug with a lid if you don't have a teapot. A lid preserves the steam while the infusion steeps – the steam contains the volatile oils which are responsible for the medicinal effect.

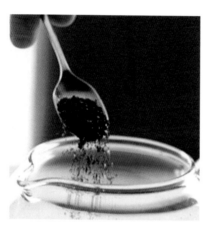

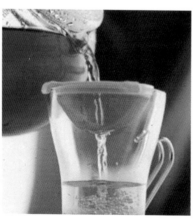

Especially suitable for Red clover (page 39), Chamomile (pages 57, 58), Red raspberry leaf (page 71), Fennel (page 96), Catnip (page 110), Lime flower (page 123)

The infusion method

For a cup
1 tsp dried or 2 tsp fresh herbs
250 ml water

For a pot
20 g dried or 30 g fresh herbs
500 ml water

Warm the cup or pot and bring fresh water to the boil. While the water is boiling, add the herbs to the warmed cup or pot.

Once the water has boiled, pour over the herbs and cover with a saucer or lid.

Allow the brew to infuse for 5–10 minutes, then strain into a cup or jug. The infusion is now ready to drink or use. If you wish to store the strained infusion, cover and refrigerate.

Keeps for 24 hours in the refrigerator.

CAUTION Don't drink any infusions during the first trimester. Don't drink more than 2 cups (500 ml) per day and vary the type.

A CREAM

Emulsions of oil and water, creams are used as a method of delivering herbs or essential oils to, or through, the skin. Once you've got used to blending the two elements (they can easily separate during the mixing stage), creams are very easy to make and much more satisfying to use than shop-bought products. The water content evaporates on the skin, which is cooling, hence the former name 'cold cream'. The easiest way to add the herb element is, as here, by using an infused oil.

Especially suitable for Rose (page 26)

The cream method

12 g beeswax, grated
125 ml herb-infused oil (see page 14)
125 ml rosewater or other hydrosol (see box, page 9)
1 vitamin E capsule

Place the beeswax into a heatproof bowl and suspend it over a pan of simmering water; add the oil and stir until all the wax has dissolved into the oil.

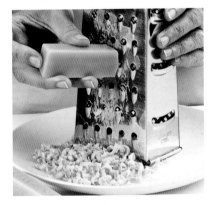

Remove the bowl from the heat and pour the contents into a clean, cool bowl. Whisk as it cools and solidifies.

Add the rosewater little by little, whisking all the time until well blended – this can take up to 2 minutes and you may need to put the bowl back over the pan to heat the mixture a little. Try not to stir in too much air. Squeeze the contents of the capsule into the mixture and stir.

Spoon into a 250 ml sterilised glass jar using a spatula and leave the cream to cool before putting on the lid to prevent condensation settling inside the lid (this can cause mould to form). Label and date, then store in the refrigerator.

Keeps for Up to 3 months in the refrigerator. When chilled, this cream becomes truly a 'cold cream'. To restore its more viscous texture, warm a little between your palms before use.

AN OINTMENT

Unlike creams, oil-based ointments or salves contain no water, and are therefore more suited to delivering helpful herbs to soothe skin conditions irritated by moisture, such as nappy rash. As they also form a protective barrier layer over the skin, ointment bases are also suitable as balms for chapped lips. The easiest way to add the herb element is, as here, by using an infused oil.

This recipe makes an ointment with a fairly loose consistency, which can be smeared over rashes and inflamed skin. It is safe because it contains no petrochemicals. Most commercial products are made with a base of petroleum jelly or paraffin wax.

Especially suitable for Pot marigold (page 93), Honey (page 106), Olive (page 116)

The ointment method

30 g beeswax, grated
250 ml herb-infused oil (see page 14)

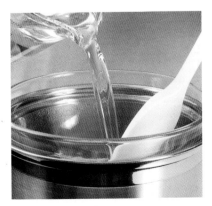

Place the beeswax into a heatproof bowl and suspend it over a pan of simmering water. Add the oil and stir until all the wax has dissolved into the oil. (If the recipe requires honey or essential oils, add it at this point.)

Remove the bowl from the heat, and while the mixture is still liquid, pour it into a 250 ml sterilised, shallow, dark glass jar. Leave to cool before putting on the lid to prevent condensation settling inside the lid (this can cause mould to grow and spoil the ointment). If the final product seems too runny or too solid, reheat and add either more beeswax or oil. Label and date, then store in a cool, dark place. Because it doesn't contain water, an ointment keeps well outside the refrigerator.

Keeps for Up to 3 months.

A DECOCTION

Similar to an infusion in that the medicinal properties of the herbs are extracted in boiling water, a decoction involves simmering herbs in water for a longer period of time. It is suitable for the woodier parts of plants, such as the roots, twigs, bark and berries. However, if you include any leaves and flowers, either add the greener material at the end, once the decoction is cooling, or pour the decoction over the leaves and flowers in a teapot or jug and allow to infuse.

Drink a decoction as a tea – either hot or cold, use externally as a toner or wash for the skin, or soak a cloth in it and use to sponge the skin or as a compress.

Especially suitable for Oats (page 37), Thyme (page 121)

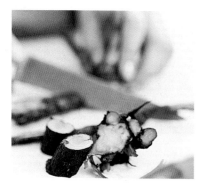

CAUTION Don't drink any decoctions during the first trimester. Don't drink more than 2 cups (500 ml) per day and vary the type.

The decoction method

20 g dried or 40 g fresh herbs
750 ml cold water

Clean the herbs by removing any dirt or foreign matter; roughly chop woody parts. Place the herbs in a saucepan with the water and bring to the boil over a medium heat.

Reduce the heat and simmer for 20–30 minutes, until the liquid has reduced by about a third (to 500 ml).

Strain the decoction through a sieve into a jug, cover and allow to cool. The decoction is ready to use, either hot or cold. Once cool, store in the refrigerator.

Keeps for 48 hours in the refrigerator.

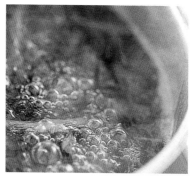

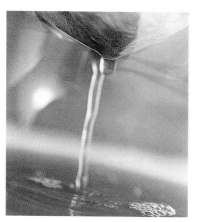

A TINCTURE

Unlike water-based remedies, tinctures can remain active for years if stored well and can be stronger in action than an infusion or decoction. Because tinctures are made by soaking herbs in alcohol to extract their active ingredients, the recipes using tinctures in this book are for external use only during pregnancy, for example, as room or linen sprays. After childbirth, diluted tinctures can be applied as compresses (see opposite) or used in perineal sprays.

The amount of herb to alcohol in a tincture is expressed as a ratio: for example 1:5 denotes one part herb (say 1 g) to five parts alcohol (5 ml).

Especially suitable for Arnica (page 89), Pot marigold (page 92)

The tincture method

200 g dried or 300 g fresh herbs
1 litre vodka or white rum (40 per cent proof)

Clean the herbs by removing any dirt or foreign matter without submerging them in water, then dry completely. Chop into thin slices or small pieces, discarding any damaged parts.

CAUTION Only use 'drinking' alcohol, such as vodka or white rum, to make tinctures. Don't take any tinctures by mouth during the first trimester. Thereafter, if taking by mouth, dilute in a little warm water or fruit juice before meals.

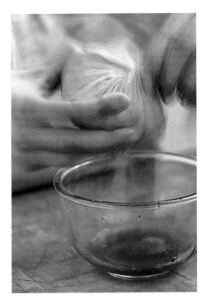

Place the chopped herbs into a large (1 litre), clean glass jar with a lid (Kilner-style preserving jar is perfect) and pour over the alcohol, making sure that it covers every part of the herb. Put on the lid, label and date the jar, then shake well and store in a cool, dark place for at least 2 and up to 6 weeks. Shake every other day.

Secure a jelly bag (see page 7) in a glass jug so that it sits above the bottom of the jug. Open the stored jar and pour the herbs and alcohol into the bag. Squeeze the jelly bag to extract as much of the tincture as possible, then discard the plant matter.

Pour the tincture, using a funnel if necessary, into two 500 ml sterilised dark glass bottles, put on the lids, label with the strength of tincture (here 1:5) and date, then store in a cool dark place until needed.

Keeps for Up to 2 years.

A COMPRESS

Compresses are a simple means of applying an infusion, decoction or diluted tincture to the skin. A cold compress can be used to soothe inflammation, reduce bruising, cool a fever or ease a headache. Use a hot compress to soothe muscle strain or ease a chest cold or sore throat.

Especially suitable for Lavender (page 74), Rescue Remedy (page 85), Arnica (page 90), Pot marigold (page 92), Catnip (page 109)

The compress method

500 ml hot or cold infusion or decoction, or 25 ml tincture diluted in 500 ml hot or cold water

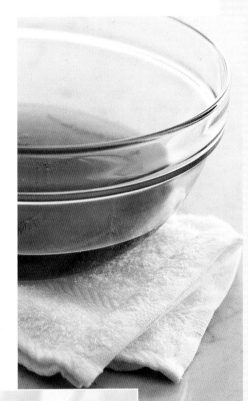

Pour the herbal liquid into a bowl and soak a clean flannel, cloth or gauze bandage in the liquid. Wring out the cloth so that it does not drip and place the compress over the affected area.

For a hot compress, re-soak and repeat when the cloth has cooled (up to 20 minutes); for a cool compress, re-soak and repeat when the cloth has become warm (up to 20 minutes).

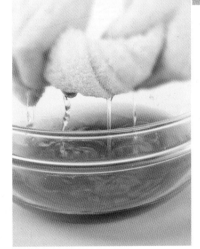

AN INFUSED OIL

When herbs are left to infuse in oil, their fat-soluble active ingredients are absorbed into the oil, making this a useful way to preserve their therapeutic properties. Strong-tasting or dried herbs and tough parts such as roots are best infused in hot oil; more leafy fresh herbs do well in the lengthier cold-infusion method.

Infused oils can be used as they are, perhaps as a massage oil or in a salad dressing or marinade, or be combined with other ingredients to make an ointment or salve (see page 11).

Extra-virgin olive oil is the best oil to use for infused oils during pregnancy – it has many medicinal properties of its own, is very good for the skin and does not turn rancid when stored. You can also cold-infuse herbs in honey or vinegar. Make sure the sterilised glass bottles and jars are completely dry when making these remedies.

Especially suitable for Lemon balm (page 30), Fennel (page 95)

Hot-infused oil method

250 g dried or 500 g fresh herbs
750 ml extra-virgin olive oil

Clean the herbs by removing any dirt or foreign matter without submerging them in water, then dry completely. Chop into thin slices or small pieces, discarding any damaged parts.

Place the chopped herbs in a heatproof glass bowl and suspend it over a pan of simmering water. Add the olive oil, cover and simmer gently for 3 hours. Check the water every 30 minutes or so, and top up, if necessary, to prevent the pan from boiling dry.

Secure a jelly bag (see page 7) in a glass jug so that it sits above the bottom of the jug. Pour the infused oil and herbs into the bag. Once cool enough to handle, squeeze the jelly bag to extract as much of the infused oil as possible then discard the plant matter.

Pour the infused oil, using a funnel if necessary, into two 500 ml sterilised dark glass bottles and put on the lids. Label and date, and store in a cool, dark place.

Keeps for Up to 6 months in a cool, dark place.

Cold-infused oil method

250 g dried or 500 g fresh herbs
750 ml–1 litre extra-virgin olive oil

Clean and dry the herbs (as for hot-infused method, left) then place the chopped herbs into a 1litre glass jar (Kilner-style preserving jar is perfect). Pour over enough of the olive oil to reach the top of the jar (to discourage the growth of mould), making sure that every part of the leafy material is covered. Stir around with a knife to 'pop' any air bubbles. Put on the lid and label and date. Shake the jar well and place in a sunny place (direct sunlight is best) to macerate for at least 2 and up to 6 weeks (the longer you leave it, the greater the therapeutic properties).

Secure a jelly bag (see page 7) in a glass jug so that it sits above the bottom of the jug. Pour the infused oil and herbs into the bag. Discard the plant matter and pour the oil back into the glass jar and replace the lid. Store in a cool, place for another week – any water will settle at the base of the jar. Decant the oil into two 500 ml sterilised dark glass bottles, using a funnel, if necessary, leaving any watery liquid at the bottom of the jar. Label the bottles and store in a cool, dark place.

Keeps for Up to a year in a cool, dark place. In cool temperatures (lower than 1.6°C or 35°F), olive oil becomes firm and will not pour; simply hold the bottle for a few minutes or rub it between your palms – the warmth will return the oil to a liquid state.

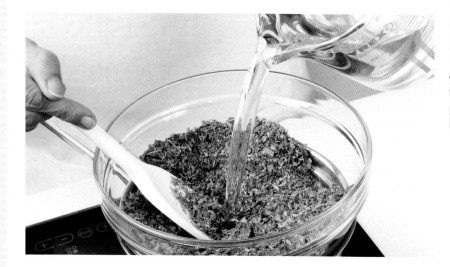

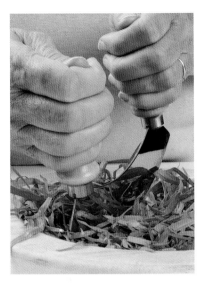

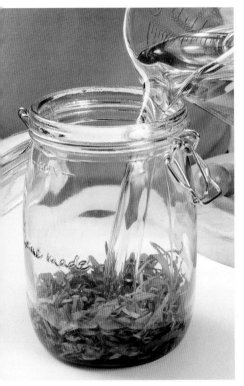

Tip For extra potency when making a cold-infused oil, repeat the process using the first infusion to infuse a new batch of the same herb.

A SYRUP

Herbal syrups gain their soothing properties partly from their sweet coating of sugar or honey – indeed the honey itself has many medicinal qualities. They are a traditional remedy for sore throats and coughs. All the syrups in this book are made using long infusions rather than tinctures, which are more potent but are made using alcohol. Be sure to use bottles with corks rather than lids or screwtops when making syrups: if the brew ferments, a cork will be pushed out while a lid or screwtop could cause the bottle to explode.

Syrups can be taken by the teaspoon – as a cough or sore-throat linctus, for example – or diluted with water and drunk as a cordial.

Especially suitable for Rosehip (page 26), Garlic (page 50), Catnip (page 111), Thyme (page 120)

The syrup method

500 ml infusion, infused for 15 minutes (see page 10) or decoction, simmered for 30 minutes (see page 12)
500 g sugar or honey

Pour the infusion or decoction into a large saucepan, add the sugar or honey and bring to the boil over a medium heat. Reduce the heat and allow to simmer, uncovered, until the mixture thickens and becomes syrupy in consistency. Remove from the heat and allow to cool.

Using a funnel, pour the liquid into two 500 ml sterilised dark glass bottles and cork. Label and date, then store in a cool, dark place. Once opened, refrigerate.

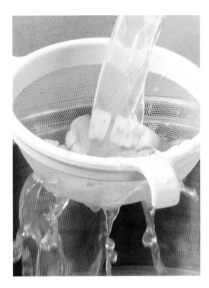

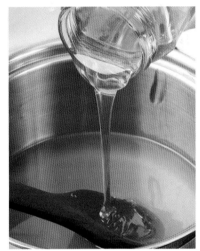

Keeps for Up to 6 months in a cool, dark place.

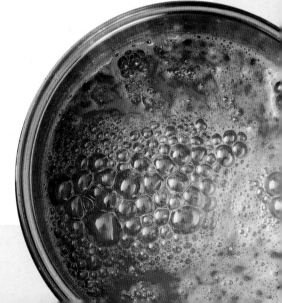

BEAUTYCARE PREPARATIONS

The recipes in this book include toners (often nothing more complicated than a simple infusion), and skin softening and renewing masks and scrubs. These rely for their effect on the emollient and astringent qualities of individual herbs combined with the drawing and tightening properties of the clay or the exfoliant powers of the oats, chickpeas, milk or almonds that form the base of the products. Because beautycare products tend to be washed off, they don't deliver the herbs' active ingredients into the bloodstream, which may be an advantage if you have lingering concerns about the safety aspects of using herbs while pregnant.

The mask recipe contains dried bentonite clay which, when it dries on the skin, draws out impurities while imparting its blend of minerals and vitamins. This is useful if you suffer from spots or rashes in pregnancy and after the birth if you feel in need of a freshening facial. If you like, you can add 1 tsp honey for its moisturising and healing properties and/or 1 tsp of olive, argan or grapeseed oil if you have very dry skin.

Especially suitable for masks Red clover (page 21), Apple (page 65), Seaweed (page 69), Honey (page 105)
Especially suitable for scrubs Oats (page 37), Chickpea (page 43)

CAUTION During pregnancy, do not use whole body masks or scrubs; these recipes make enough for the face, feet or hands only.

The mask method

2 tbsp bentonite clay
2–3 tbsp herbal infusion (see page 10) or hydrosol (see box, page 9)

Place the dried clay in a ceramic or glass bowl, stir in enough of the infusion or hydrosol to make a smooth paste, mixing well to smooth out lumps. Keep stirring until you have the desired consistency.

Using your fingers, apply the mask to cleansed skin, avoiding the eye and mouth areas, then lie down and relax for 10–15 minutes as the mask dries. Splash off the mask with warm water, and wipe away the vestiges with cottonwool soaked in rosewater.

Keeps for Not suitable for storing.

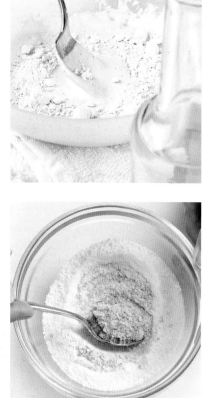

The scrub method

1 tbsp fine oatmeal, ground almonds or gram (chickpea) flour
1 tbsp milk powder
2–3 tbsp herbal infusion (see page 10) or hydrosol (see box, page 9)

Mix the dry ingredients together in a ceramic or glass bowl, then blend to a paste using as much of the infusion or hydrosol as desired.

Moisten the skin, then massage in the scrub, making circles with your fingertips in an outward direction all over the area.

Splash off the scrub with warm water or wipe away with a warm wet flannel, then splash with cool water.

Keeps for Not suitable for storing.

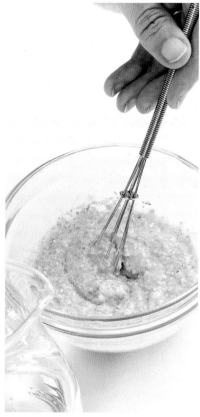

HERBAL BATHS

In a warm bath muscles relax and blood vessels dilate, improving peripheral circulation and giving the immune and waste-disposal systems a boost. Skin softened by warm water absorbs essential oils and herbal ingredients efficiently. You can add leaves, flowers and seeds directly to the bath or make an infusion (see page 10) to pour in.

During pregnancy, plunging your feet into cool water up to the knees brings relief to aching feet and puffy ankles.

Hydrotherapists and naturopaths recommend sitz baths (simply immersing your lower half in water) to relieve pain or infection in the pelvic area. Sitz baths can be incredibly soothing in the postnatal period. Start 24 hours after the birth to ease perineal swelling, bruising and pain.

The heat of steam facials can be useful, occasionally, too. As blood vessels in the skin dilate and sweat glands produce perspiration, the increased blood flow allows waste products to pass out to skin cells to be eliminated and the skin to take up nutrients and oxygen from the blood. They can also clear blocked sinuses, relax tense muscles in the neck and shoulders, and deepen the breathing for increased relaxation at stressful times.

CAUTION During pregnancy: keep the water temperature less than 30–35°C (85–95°F). If you feel too hot during a steam facial treatment, stop immediately.

Tip Sip water to rehydrate the body as you bathe – this can help to relieve symptoms as varied as headaches, ill temper and constipation.

Especially suitable for baths Rose (page 26), Oats (page 37), Seaweed (page 69), Lavender (page 73), Pot marigold (page 92)

Especially suitable for steams Nettle (page 29), Fennel (page 96), Lime flower (page 123)

The oil bath method

2 tsp carrier oil, such as olive or grapeseed oil
2 drops essential oil, optional

If using essential oil, mix with the carrier oil in a small glass or ceramic bowl to ensure the essential oil is safely diluted before use.

Stir the diluted oils on to the surface of the bathwater after turning off the taps and just before stepping in. Be prepared to clean the oily film from the bath after use.

Keeps for Not suitable for storing.

The sitz bath method

Herbal infusion or essential oils (see individual recipes)

Fill a portable sitz bath, plastic basin or bucket, or half-fill the bath with water. Pour in the herbal remedy or diluted essential oils, if using, and swish well with your fingers to disperse.

Sit in the water, soaking your pelvic region for up to 20 minutes. Repeat several times a day.

MASSAGE BLENDS

Massage using herbal oils delivers the benefits of the active ingredients in the herbs, and the nutrients and brain-friendly fats in the oils. It can be amazingly comforting during pregnancy, especially if your skin is feeling tight or itchy. Massage is also an effective way to ease tense muscles and calm racing thoughts. It gives the immune and waste-disposal systems a boost too.

During labour, pressure-point massage on the sacrum at the base of the spine can help to keep you focused – ask your midwife or a natural birth practitioner for advice well in advance so you can teach your birth partner what to do.

If you feel like a full-body or aromatherapy massage during pregnancy, it's best to find a qualified professional who specialises in pregnancy, but it's safe to have a partner or friend ease out tight muscles in your shoulders, and aches and tiredness in your feet and hands. Ask for a lower back and shoulder massage after work or before bed.

Tip As your bump grows, the safest and most comfortable position to receive a back or shoulder massage is kneeling on a folded blanket and leaning forwards on to a large pile of cushions.

Especially suitable for Lavender (page 74), Neroli (page 82), Jasmine (page 101), Catnip (page 111)

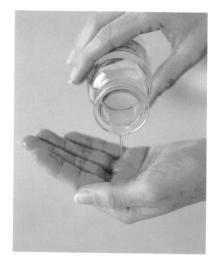

The pregnancy massage blend

2 tsp carrier oil, such as olive or grapeseed oil
2 drops essential oil, optional

If using essential oil, mix with the carrier oil in a small glass or ceramic bowl to ensure the essential oils are safely diluted before use. These proportions make an especially low dilution suitable for pregnancy.

Warm a little of the oil between both palms before applying to the skin – just enough so that the hands slide comfortably over the skin. Reapply oil when the hands start to drag.

Keeps for Not suitable for storing.

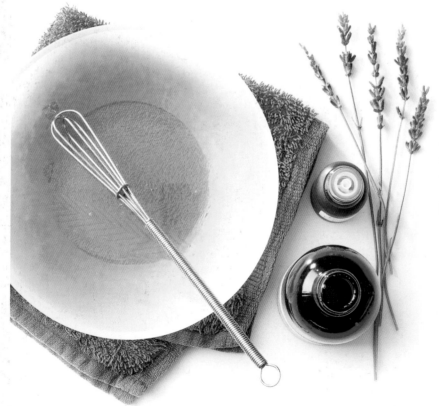

Part 2
FERTILITY-BOOSTING HERBS

Herbs to detox and nourish, balance the hormones
and calm the nerves in the pre-conception months; stop taking
these herbs immediately you suspect you might be pregnant

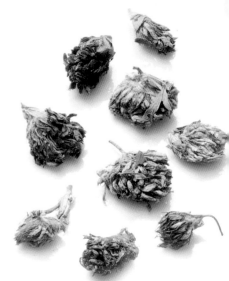

Red clover

fertility tonic, purifying

Red clover is a lucky charm, bringing blessings. In Celtic lore, the shamrock (*seamrog* translates as 'cloverlet') is a symbol of mother earth and her womanly essence. Traditionally, an Irish wedding bouquet contains red clover for fertility and good fortune.

CAUTION Avoid if you have a history of breast cancer, uterine fibroids or endometriosis, or are taking birth-control or fertility drugs. Red clover can interfere with blood-thinning drugs.

The pretty reddish-pink flowers of the meadow plant red, or wild, clover (*Trifolium pratense*) are one of the richest sources of isoflavones, phytoestrogens or plant chemicals that act on the body like the reproductive hormone oestrogen, but in a milder form. American fertility herbalist Susun Weed calls it the single best aid to fertility after the age of forty.

This herb has long been used for its purifying – and detoxifying – action. It supports the liver, improves circulation, acts as an expectorant and has a diuretic action. Red clover is also used to soothe skin conditions such as eczema and rashes. The flowering tops are nutrient-rich and a good source of antioxidant vitamin C, B vitamins, and the useful minerals for fertility, calcium and magnesium.

PLANT TIPS

❋ Harvest the flowers early in the morning while they are still covered in dew. You can pick throughout the growing season, but they are at their best from mid-spring to early summer. Pick blooms that are fully open, but not yet brown.

USING THE HERB

To make the vagina more sperm-friendly, make a tea, using 1 tsp of the dried flowers in a mug (200 ml) of boiled water. Steep for 30 minutes. Drink 2 or 3 cups a day.

In cooking, evidence suggests adding young leaves to salads (see opposite) may bring nutritional benefits, but their medicinal properties have not been well studied. You can also cook the leaves as you would spinach. To add a vanilla-like perfume and flavour to cakes, crumble dried leaves into the batter. The taste works well with maple syrup and almonds.

OFF-THE-SHELF REMEDIES

❋ Take 3–5 ml (1:5) tincture three times a day to detox and boost intake of nutrients.
❋ Ointments containing 10–15 per cent flowerheads are recommended to treat skin rashes; apply direct to the affected area.
❋ A fluid extract (1:1) can be used to bathe rough or itchy skin.
❋ Dr Hauschka Regenerating range skincare products use an extract of organic whole red clover for its antioxidant properties and to encourage skin renewal.
❋ Choose smudging herbs (herbs

that can be burned for their purifying effect) containing red clover to cleanse your home.

Red clover infusion

Make this fertility aid the evening before you drink it, refrigerate until needed and make a new batch every other day. To reduce the tannic taste, add a handful of lemon balm, mint or chamomile.

30 g dried red clover flowers
1 litre freshly boiled water
honey or maple syrup, to taste

Place the flowers in a warmed teapot or jug and pour over the water. Put on a lid. Steep for at least 4 hours, but preferably overnight, before straining. Sweeten to taste and, on hot days, drink over ice or with a slice of lemon.

Red clover and honey clay mask

Combine the cleansing properties of red clover with clay in a clarifying mask to soothe the skin and help you relax: relaxation is one of the surest ways to make pregnancy more likely.

2 tbsp bentonite clay
2 tbsp red clover infusion (see above)
2 tsp runny honey
2 tsp rosewater or hydrosol, plus extra for cleansing
½ tsp rosehip or argan oil

Place the dried clay in a ceramic or glass bowl, stir in the infusion and honey, mixing well until smooth. Apply the mask to cleansed skin using your fingers, avoiding the eye and mouth areas, then relax for 10–15 minutes as the mask dries.

Splash off the mask with warm water, and wipe away the vestiges with cottonwool soaked in rosewater. Moisturise with a little nourishing rosehip or argan oil.

Fertility leaf salad

Clover leaves and flowers make a pretty addition to a springtime salad. Spinach leaves contain protein in addition to good amounts of fertility-friendly vitamins and minerals, including folate. The cheese in this recipe

contributes calcium and the walnuts omega-3 fatty acids, vital for healthy functioning of the reproductive system.

SERVES 2

25 g lamb's leaf lettuce
75 g baby spinach leaves
handful of red clover leaves
50 g walnuts, halved and toasted
100 g goat's cheese, broken into bite-sized pieces
1 tbsp fresh chives, snipped
handful of red clover flowers

For the dressing
1 tsp cider vinegar
1 tsp walnut oil
2 tbsp extra-virgin olive oil
1 tsp runny honey or ½ tsp maple syrup
½ lemon
½ tsp Dijon mustard
black pepper and sea salt, to taste

Wash and spin dry the leaves, then toss in a bowl with the toasted walnuts and cheese pieces. Add the chives and clover flowers.

To make the dressing, whisk together the vinegar and oils, then stir in the honey or maple syrup, a squeeze of lemon juice and the mustard. Season to taste, and toss add to the salad.

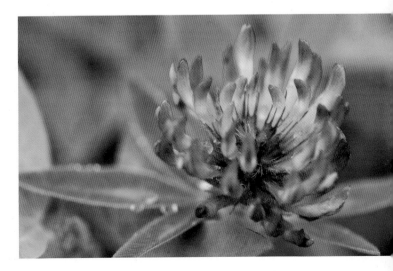

Chasteberry

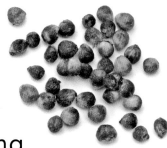

hormone-balancing, sustaining

This is one of the oldest known herbs with a medicinal reputation for menstrual problems. The berries were used in ancient times in rites to venerate Demeter or Ceres, the Greek and Roman goddesses of growth in the natural world, or mother nature.

The fruit of the chaste tree is perhaps the best-known herbal fertility-enhancer. Chasteberry (*Vitex agnus castus*) does not contain hormones, but it acts on the hypothalamus and pituitary gland, which control the hormonal system. The herb seems to stimulate and regulate the production of the hormones that govern the menstrual cycle. Chasteberry also seems to help women with amenorrhoea, the absence of periods, and encourages production of the most important hormone in sustaining pregnancy, progesterone.

Progesterone levels rise at ovulation and keep on rising in the second half of the menstrual cycle to maintain a pregnancy. At the same time, it inhibits the release of prolactin, which can adversely affect fertility. This herb may also increase production of luteinising hormone (LH), which aids conception, and decrease levels of follicle-stimulating hormone (FSH), high levels of which make conception less likely.

Based on preliminary trials, the medical community regards this herb as safe, well-tolerated and possibly effective for fertility disorders. In Germany, it is approved for use to treat menstrual irregularities and PMS and is prescribed by doctors for fertility problems connected with insufficient levels of progesterone in the second half of the menstrual cycle. It may also be useful for rebalancing your hormones if you've recently stopped taking birth-control pills.

CAUTION Avoid if taking birth-control or fertility drugs, synthetic progesterone or HRT, and during IVF treatment. Do not use if you have a history of breast cancer. If taking antipsychotic drugs, talk to your doctor to check suitabililty.

PLANT TIPS

❋ This is not a herb you can harvest easily yourself – remedies are made from the dried ripe dark-purple seeds, or berries, which in early autumn resemble peppercorns (the herb is also known as monk's pepper or wild pepper).

USING THE HERB

To enhance fertility, persistence is the key to the effectiveness of chasteberry. It is slow-acting and has a cumulative rather than an immediate effect. Take the tea or capsules for at least three menstrual cycles, though changes may not be evident until after six months. Some herbalists and doctors recommend taking it for 12–18 months without a break; others recommend taking a break during menstruation. Consult a herbalist for advice.

Take chasteberry at the same time every day, as you would a birth-control pill. Early morning is best. If you find this makes you feel tired, switch to the evening.

To reduce the spiciness or slight aftertaste of chasteberry tea, grate a little fresh ginger root into the cup before pouring over boiling water, or combine with green tea.

OFF-THE-SHELF REMEDIES

❋ The daily dose of the dried ground herb used in many clinical trials is 20–40 mg, taken in capsule form. Other trials used a liquid extract (1:5, 25 per cent alcohol), with 40 drops taken each morning. Doctors might prescribe much higher (400–500 mg) daily doses for a short time. Because every woman's hormone levels differ, it's best to have a dose prescribed by a herbalist.

❋ When searching for fertility supplements containing chasteberry, look for the name 'vitex'. Supplements may also include red clover (see page 20). In one study of women taking a supplement combining chasteberry with an extract of green tea and folic acid, a third became pregnant within five months compared with none in the group taking a placebo.

❋ Buy products stating on the label that the amount is 'standardised', meaning it contains a defined amount of active ingredients, 0.6 per cent agnoside.

IN THE GARDEN

This lilac-like shrub is native to the Mediterranean and western Asia, and has scented foliage and attractive mauve to deep-purple flowers from late summer. These attract bees and butterflies, making the plant a pretty addition to the back of a sunny border. It is a riverbank plant, preferring wet conditions, and requires frost protection in spring. To encourage the attractive red berries to develop, don't overwater while the flowers are forming.

❋ The homeopathic remedy agnus castus is prescribed for lack of libido and accompanying depression, anxiety or exhaustion, lack of energy or forgetfulness as well as infertility and menstrual problems. It is also available in the homeopathic preparation Memorin to encourage mental alertness.

❋ The Moroccan spice blend ras el hanout traditionally includes chasteberries alongside cardamom, nutmeg, ginger and other spices.

❋ Chasteberry extract can be found in some brands labelled as 'women's teas', blended to support the menstrual cycle – try the Yogi Tea Woman's Moon Cycle®.

Chasteberry tea

If you can source dried berries, you might like to make a tea yourself rather than relying on teabags. The flavour is spicy and perfumed, rather reminiscent of peppermint. Chasteberry tea is said to increase libido.

1 tsp dried chasteberries
200 ml freshly boiled water
honey, to taste

Place the dried berries in a pot and pour over the water. Allow to steep for 10 minutes, then strain into a mug and sweeten with honey, if desired.

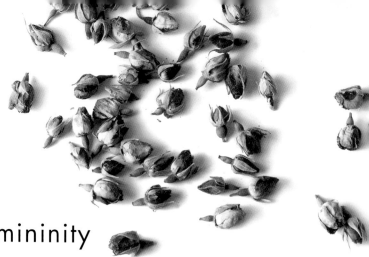

Rose

uplifting, nurturing femininity

If a pregnant woman chooses a rose when offered a lily and a rose, she is said to be carrying a girl.

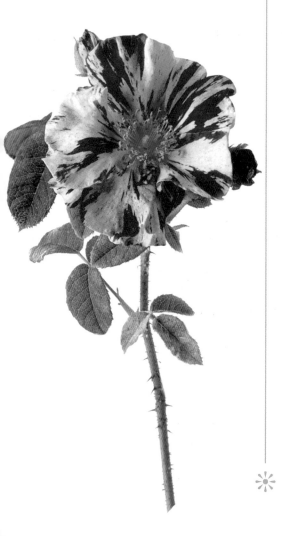

The 'queen of flowers' has been cultivated for some 3,000 years and is valued for its intensely scented essential oil, petals and hips. The petals are said to be especially beneficial for the female reproductive system. Essential oil of rose (*Rosa centifolia* or *R. damascena*) is calming and lifts the spirits. It is useful in the months before conception for quelling anxiety, easing the effects of stress and promoting rest.

Rose essential oil is used by aromatherapists to treat PMS and balance the menstrual cycle, and to deepen feelings of femininity and sexuality. It is also gently restorative for sensitive and inflamed skin, having a purifying, strengthening and lifting action. In the preconception months, the essential oil works well with geranium (for hormonal balance), neroli (for peacefulness and its aphrodisiac properties) and bergamot (to counter frustration).

Rose petals (*R. rugosa* or *R. gallica*) have been prepared as an astringent rosewater (the tannins in the plant give this action) since the time of the Arab physician Ibn Sina (980–1037). The red hips of the dog rose (*R. canina*) are a good source of vitamin C, calcium and iron, which are important during pregnancy. They also have a gently laxative and diuretic effect. In Traditional Chinese Medicine their relative, R. *laevigata*, is prescribed to regulate the menstrual cycle.

PLANT TIPS

* Only pick roses you have grown yourself – raise the *R. rugosa* or *R. gallica* cultivars. Do not use roses from florists or garden centres, which are likely to have been treated with pesticides.
* Pick rosehips from the hedgerows when deep red in autumn, avoiding those that have basked all summer in exhaust fumes.
* When gathering petals, pick them as close to dawn as you can when the life force within the dew-drenched plant is supposedly most potent then. By mid-morning, the essential oil content of rose petals plummets by 40 per cent.

CAUTION Avoid essential oil of rose in the first trimester.

USING THE HERB

For tired eyes, relax for 10 minutes with chilled rose petals over your eyes.

For calming the nerves, detoxing and menstrual problems, drink rose petal tea. Either steep 1 tsp dried petals with 200 ml just-boiled water for 5–10 minutes or measure ½ cup of fresh petals, place in a pan with 2 cups water, bring to the boil and simmer (covered) for 5 minutes. Strain into a cup; sweeten with honey, if desired. Alternatively, relax in a rose-scented bath (see page 26).

If you feel under the weather or in the early stages of a cold, rosehip tea makes a useful immune-boosting pick-me-up. Pour 200 ml boiling water over 1 tsp chopped dried hips and allow to steep for at least 5 minutes. Alternatively, take some rose-hip syrup (see page 26).

As a skin treatment for thread veins, make a mask of 1 tbsp dried rose petals pounded in a pestle and mortar and mixed with 1 tbsp set honey and a little natural yogurt. Apply to the skin, relax for 15 minutes, then wash off with cool water. Or try cold cream (see page 26) to keep hands looking their best.

OFF-THE-SHELF REMEDIES

❋ Essential oil of rose can be used in a massage oil to build self-confidence and hope, counter fear, regret or worries about the past and ease feelings of grief or lack of conviction about a decision. Use 10 drops of essential oil to 50 ml of carrier oil. If you feel exhausted or fearful of change, ask your partner to massage your feet with 5 drops of essential oil of rose mixed into 1 tbsp of sweet almond oil.

❋ Rosewater is an effective toner for delicate or dry skin; opt for a 'hydrosol' (see box, page 9). It contains many of the plant's therapeutic properties. You also can soak a hot flannel in it, and apply the wrung-out cloth to your forehead for tension headaches or over your eyes after a weeping session.

❋ A little 100 per cent rosa mosqueta oil from Chile or Argentina massaged into your face twice daily can help to prevent sun damage and chloasma.

BUYING ROSE OIL

Otto or attar of rose, steam-distilled from the petals, is the best-quality essential oil and has the greatest therapeutic value. It crystallises at room temperature (simply hold the bottle for a few minutes and the warmth of your hands will return the oil to liquid form). Essential oil of rose is among the most costly of oils – Turkish (from Esparta) or Bulgarian (from the Valley of the Roses near Kazanlik) oils are top quality. Beware cheap rose oils, which are likely to have been adulterated, or 'extended', often with geranium or palmarosa oils. For a cheaper rose oil, look for 5 per cent dilutions of the essential oil in a base oil. Rose absolute, extracted using a solvent, is a less costly oil, more suited to perfumery.

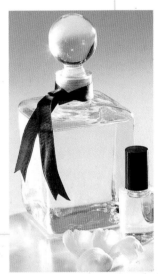

❋ The Bach Flower Remedy Rock Rose© is recommended if you feel overcome by fear of motherhood – take 2 drops in a glass of water. It is also a constituent of Rescue Remedy© (see page 85), useful for crises at every stage of pregnancy. Wild Rose© can help if you have a sense of drifting through life.

LOOKING AHEAD Later on in pregnancy, oil of rosa mosqueta rosehips from the Andes (*R. affinis rubiginosa*) has remarkable skin-repair properties thanks to its essential fatty acids. In addition to reducing sun damage and hyper-pigmentation, these can soften visible signs of stretchmarks and/or surgical scar tissue. Favour belly butters and stretchmark creams that contain rosehip oil and 2–4 weeks before a planned caesarean, rub rosehip oil into the incision area to prevent scar formation. Continue after the stitches have been removed and the area has healed.

Cold cream

Cold creams have a cooling effect on the skin. Use on the hands, massaging it in well to release its calming scent. You will need a 60 ml sterilised glass jar with a lid.

10 g beeswax, grated
2 tbsp olive oil
1 tbsp rosewater or hydrosol
10 drops essential oil of rose
2 drops essential oil of frankincense

Place the beeswax into a heatproof bowl. Suspend over a pan of simmering water, add the olive oil and stir until all the wax has dissolved into the oil. Remove the bowl from the heat, pour the contents into another, cool, bowl, and whisk as it cools and solidifies.

Add the rosewater drop by drop, whisking all the time until well blended; you may need to put the bowl back over the pan to reheat the mixture. Stir in the essential oils and spoon into the jar. Once it has cooled, put on the lid. Store in the refrigerator for up to three months.

Rosehip syrup

As well as being a traditional remedy for chest infections and coughs, this syrup can be drizzled over ice-cream and yogurt, rice pudding, porridge and pancakes, and used to sweeten tea. You will need a 750 ml sterilised glass preserving bottle with a lid or stopper.

500 g rosehips, topped, tailed and washed well
1.5 litres water
250 g sugar
1 tbsp rosewater
juice of 1 lemon

Roughly chop the hips and place them in a large pan with 1 litre of the water. Bring to the boil, then simmer for 15–20 minutes, until soft. Strain through a muslin-lined sieve, catching the juice in a large bowl. Set the bowl aside. Put the pulp back in the pan and add another 500 ml of water. Bring to the boil, then strain through the muslin again into the same bowl. This time discard the pulp.

Pour all the juice into the pan, bring to the boil and allow to simmer until reduced by half. Add the sugar and

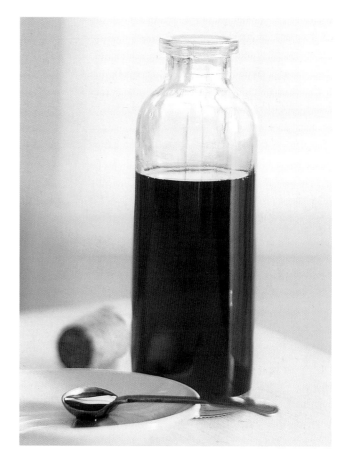

boil rapidly for 5 minutes, skimming off any scum. Finally, stir in the rosewater and lemon juice. Using a funnel, fill the bottle, label and date, and store in a cool, dark place. Once opened, refrigerate; this keeps for up to six months.

Rose petal and milk bath bag

A rose-scented bath is good for exhaustion and lifts the spirits. Follow with a voluptuous rose body oil – mix 6 drops of essential oil of rose into 2 tbsp of grapeseed oil.

25 g dried rose petals
6 tbsp milk powder
6 drops essential oil of rose

Pound the rose petals using a pestle and mortar until reduced to dust. Place the milk powder and rose petals in the centre of a large square of muslin, drop on the essential oil, and tie to secure. Float in the water as the bath runs, then step in and relax in the silky scented water.

Nettle

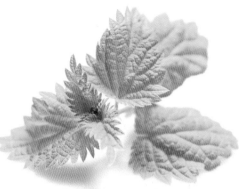

nourishing, cleansing

Nettles are associated with fertility because their shoots are the first signs of life after winter. Their green hue – a result of high amounts of chlorophyll, which sustains plant life – is further evidence of their life-giving essence.

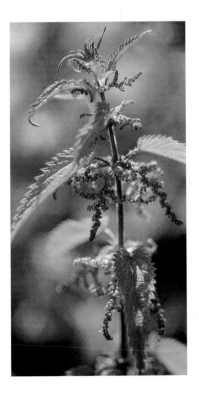

You might be inclined to avoid the sharp-toothed leaves and downy-needled stems of the stinging nettle *Urtica dioica*, but this is one of the finest natural fertility tonics – and available for free in most parts of the world. This common weed is among the most nutritious of plants and has a long history as a pot herb and tonic for anaemia. Studies show that that getting plenty of nutrient-dense fresh food in the preconception period can boost fertility.

Nettles are packed with the most easily absorbed plant form of iron and contain calcium (most mums-to-be don't get enough of either in their diet), as well as the pre-conception musts folate, vitamin C, protein, potassium and magnesium. This herb also contains beta-carotene (necessary during intense periods of cell growth) and vitamin K (for strong bones and to reduce the risk of nausea).

Nettle leaves have a diuretic action, which is why they are often found in detox preparations, and are both stimulating and restorative for the kidneys and bladder. The herb is also a blood-purifier, promotes sweating and cleanses the respiratory system by loosening mucus. Nettles can treat symptoms of stress and restore vitality (the Greek poet Ovid considered the seeds a virility tonic and aphrodisiac). Chemicals in the plant are antiviral and immune stimulants. They may lessen pain by reducing levels of inflammatory chemicals and affecting how the body transmits pain signals.

PLANT TIPS
* Wear thick gloves and long sleeves when picking; it's safest to cut with scissors.
* The young shoots – up to about 15 cm in height – are most palatable for cooking. Search them out in early spring and in autumn. For cooking, you can leave them on the tender stalks.
* Older nettles are coarser in texture and should only be used for drying or making tea. They must be cooked.

CAUTION Avoid nettles if you take blood-thinning medication or diuretics, drugs for heart problems or diabetes, or anti-inflammatories.

USING THE HERB

For a fertility boost, treat nettles like spinach – cook in a covered pan with a little water. Check after a few minutes and allow to steam till tender (this may take 10–15 minutes as the shoots get older). A full pan of uncooked leaves produces only a few tablespoons of cooked leaves. You can use them in soups (see Spring soup, opposite), with eggs, on pizza, in quiches and buttered with nutmeg. Reserve the cooking liquid to add to stocks, or refrigerate and drink 1–2 tbsp daily. Freeze cooked nettles in ice-cube trays for future use.

As an energy tonic, drink the freshly squeezed juice of the young leaves. To make it more palatable, mix with carrot juice.

For oily hair or dandruff and generally for gloss and swing, a nettle conditioning rinse is an old folk remedy. Use cooled tea or the water from simmered nettles or simmer 50 g fresh nettles in 1 litre water for 15 minutes, strain and use warm.

For aching feet at the end of a long day, add 1 tbsp of nettle tincture (1:5) and 1 tbsp of cider vinegar to a footbath (see page 13 for making a tincture).

To calm itchy skin, try the facial steam opposite.

LOOKING AHEAD If you feel run down or over-tired, in pregnancy, nettle tea is a good pick-me-up after the first trimester. Use 3–4 tsp of the dried leaves to ⅔ cup of boiling water. Steep for 5 minutes. Drink 2–4 cups daily. Since this plant is a diuretic, accompany each cup of nettle tea with a glass of water.

In your birth bag, pack a flask of nettle tea; it is considered a natural painkiller and may have a sedative action.

After the birth, drink nettle tea in the days and weeks that follow to restore energy, cleanse your system and build up your supply of milk. Look out, too, for products made from nettle root, which is effective in stemming post-pregnancy hair loss.

OFF-THE-SHELF REMEDIES

※ For herbal remedies look for the variety name *Urtica dioica* – the large perennial with many medicinal uses.

※ Capsules of the freeze-dried leaf are particularly effective for the sneezing and itching associated with hayfever. This method of drying preserves the effective ingredients. Try taking 2–4 g three times daily if avoiding oral antihistamines or decongestant drugs before pregnancy or while breastfeeding.

※ Nettle tincture (1:5), 1–4 ml taken three to four times daily is a tonic, advisable if you're not eating as well as you should, or eat junk food regularly. You can make the tincture, but it's less work (and easier on the hands) to buy off the shelf.

※ Nettle teabags – as a single ingredient or part of a blend – are sold for fertility and pregnancy. Peppermint and nettle make a tasty combination if you find nettle alone too astringent. Choose organic.

※ WALA herbal remedies – preparations developed using anthrosophical principles of holistic treatment, following the philosophy of Rudolf Steiner developed in the late 19th and early 20th centuries – include a nettle preparation prescribed for problems in the pelvic region, including heavy periods and bleeding caused by uterine fibroids.

ECO FIBRE

Since earliest times nettles have been thought of as a woman's herb because they are associated with spinning. Indeed, the name is related to Latin, German and Sanskrit words meaning 'to bind'. Textiles woven from nettle stems are the latest news in eco fabric manufacture. The fabric has all the qualities of linen and is especially hard-wearing but almost as tactile as silk. Some compare the fibres to the best Egyptian cotton, yet the fabric shares the thermal qualities of pure wool, the hollow stems preserving warmth in winter and coolness in summer. Search out nettle bedlinen and clothing online.

Spring soup

The sting is neutralised when stinging nettles are cooked. Nine-herb soup is a folk remedy from northern Europe said to stimulate new life in early spring after the dormancy of winter. Make it by adding the first herbs of spring, such as mint, thyme and chives, to a nettle soup.

SERVES 2

50 g olive oil
1 large onion, chopped
1 clove garlic, chopped
300 g young nettle shoots
600 ml vegetable or chicken stock
2 medium potatoes, diced
freshly ground black pepper, to season
2 tbsp crème fraîche
few sprigs of mint, sage, rosemary or thyme, roughly chopped
small bunch of chives, chopped

In a large pan, heat the olive oil and sweat the onion and garlic. Meanwhile, put on rubber gloves and wash the nettle shoots and leaves well. Roughly chop, discarding any coarse stalks.

When the onion is soft, add the stock to the pan and bring to the boil. Turn down to a simmer and add the diced potato and chopped nettles. Allow to simmer for 10–15 minutes, or until the potatoes are just tender. Remove from the heat.

Blend to a smooth consistency, adding more stock or water if the soup seems a little thick or grainy. Season with black pepper and pour into bowls. Add a swirl of crème fraîche and a good sprinkling of the fresh herbs and chives to each.

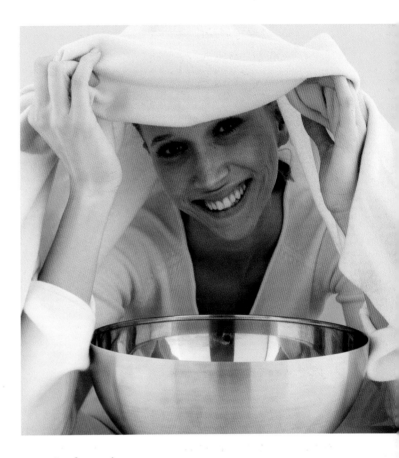

Nettle facial steam

Nettles are used to calm inflamed or itching skin. The herb has an astringent action and kills germs while healing wounds. Use this facial treatment for cleansing and clearing skin prone to hormonal outbreaks.

300 g fresh nettles
1 litre water
1 tsp grapeseed oil

Roughly chop the nettles with scissors. Place in a pan with the water, bring to the boil (covered) and simmer for 10 minutes, until the water has a green tinge.

Strain into a bowl and keeping your face about 20 cm from the water and your eyes closed, cover your head and the bowl with a large towel to trap the steam. Remain under the towel for 5–10 minutes, breathing deeply. After emerging, place a cooled wet flannel over your face and wipe away. Immediately moisturise using the grapeseed oil. If you feel lightheaded at any point, stop and lie down for 10 minutes.

Lemon balm

calming the nerves, kindling joy

In Greek mythology, Melissa was a nymph charged with nursing the baby Zeus, feeding him honey instead of milk. In other ancient texts, she is associated with the moon goddess Artemis, who brings pain relief to women in labour.

The leaves of this mint-like plant give off a distinct lemony scent when brushed, and taste of lemon, too. The botanical name, *Melissa officinalis*, derives from the Greek for 'honey bee' *melissa*, perhaps because the sweet-smelling blooms attract so many bees. Its older name, balsam, gives a good indication of its medicinal use as a soothing balm.

Lemon balm has been valued since ancient times for its ability to raise the spirits at times of emotional upset and loss, foster a sense of purpose, stimulate the brain and even renew youthfulness. The 16th-century herbalist John Gerard said it 'comforts the heart, and driveth away all melancholy and sadnesse...'. It is recommended by herbalists for the female reproductive system, to treat PMS and regulate the menstrual cycle, dissipating any nervous tension that may accompany them. Melissa's sedative ingredients make a good night's sleep more likely. This is also a good herb if you get a nervous tummy when worried or anxious. Its antispasmodic and carminative actions calm digestive disorders such as bloating, wind and cramps when it is used as a tea or in a massage oil, and aid digestion. Staying calm and getting plenty of sleep during the pre-pregnancy period promotes relaxation and turns off the body's stress reactions. This relaxation response has been shown to improve quality of life in the stressful preconception period as well as make fertility treatment more successful and improve the likelihood of conception.

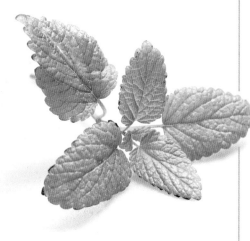

CAUTION Do not use if you are taking sedatives or thyroid medication. The essential oil is best administered by a qualified aromatherapist for a stress-relieving massage.

PLANT TIPS

❋ For best taste and scent, pick the leaves just before the plant flowers. After blooming it loses some of its sweet balminess.

❋ Like mint, whose family it shares, this herb spreads liberally – maybe one reason it is linked to fertility – so you might prefer to plant it in pots rather than a bed (and even then it will spring up everywhere).

❋ When growing melissa, cut down the stems in autumn, leaving the root to sprout again in early spring.

USING THE HERB

If you have difficulty getting to sleep or to calm frazzled nerves, have a cup of lemon balm tea in the evening: pour 200 ml of boiling water into a mug containing 1 tsp of fresh leaves and steep for 10 minutes. Strain, and sweeten with honey, if desired. Fresh leaves make a more fragrant tea than dried herbs, which can lack flavour.

To combat a cold sore in its early stages, apply cooled tea using a cotton ball.

For natural pain relief for insect bites and stings, crush a leaf and rub over the affected area.

To enhance other herbal tea blends, add lemon balm to raspberry leaf (see page 72), nettle (see page 27) and mint teas. Its delicate flavour is a favourite in chilled summer drinks (see Carmelite cup, page 32).

OFF-THE-SHELF REMEDIES

❋ The essential oil is very expensive; because it is so difficult to extract by steam-distillation, it may be 'extended' with a citrus oil or lemongrass oil. Check the label to ensure you are buying 100 per cent *Melissa officinalis*.

❋ Skincare products for sensitive skin can contain lemon balm; Dr Hauschka Melissa Day Cream and Neal's Yard Melissa Hand Cream are recommended.

❋ Capsules can be taken for insomnia or indigestion; the recommended dose is 300–500 mg three times daily.

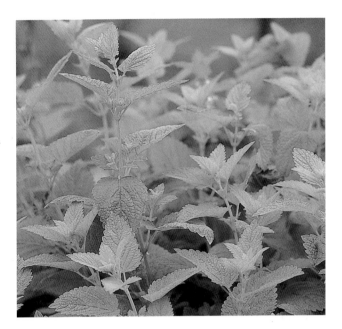

❋ Lemon balm tincture is also available; take 2–3 ml three times a day to reduce indigestion, bloating, or flatulence. Tincture can also be taken if you are having trouble sleeping.

❋ Look out for honey from bees fed on lemon balm flowers, which is rated for its fine flavour, or honey scented with sprigs of the plant.

❋ Natural air fresheners and sleep pillows often contain a mix of lemon balm, chamomile, lavender and hops – traditional blends for encouraging sleep.

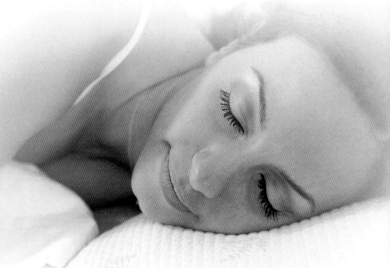

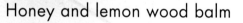

the heat and strain into a jug, either through a jelly bag or muslin-lined fine sieve. Press with the back of a wooden spoon to extract as much oil as possible. Using a funnel, pour the infused oil into the bottle, put on the lid and label. Store in a cool, dark place for up to a year.

To make the wood balm, place the beeswax, honey and 3 tbsp of the infused oil into a heatproof bowl over a pan of simmering water and stir over the heat until well combined. Stir in the essential oil. Spoon into a glass jar and allow to cool and set before using. The balm will keep for up to three months.

Carmelite cup

This iced summer drink, which calls on the cooling action of lemon balm, is based on a panacea for headaches, gastric problems and nervous tension first brewed in the 17th century by members of the Carmelite religious order in France. A secret blend of 14 therapeutic plants and nine spices, it may have resembled Chartreuse or Benedictine. The historic blend was a perfume; this recipe makes more of a spicy homemade lemonade.

SERVES 2

25 g fresh lemon balm leaves, plus extra to garnish
zest and juice of 1 large organic lemon
30 g sugar
½ cinnamon stick
3 cloves
500 ml boiling water
lemon and orange slices, to garnish
few springs of mint, to garnish
nutmeg, freshly grated

Place the lemon balm leaves, lemon zest, sugar, cinnamon stick and cloves in a heatproof jug and pour over the water. Stir until the sugar is dissolved, then cover to preserve the aromatic oils and leave to infuse until cool.

Strain, add the lemon juice and refrigerate until chilled. Serve over ice with twists of lemon and orange, sprigs of mint and lemon balm, and a grating of fresh nutmeg.

Honey and lemon wood balm

'Bee balm' as an ingredient of furniture polish is mentioned by Shakespeare. Many women trying to conceive cut down on chemical household cleaners and replace them with more eco-friendly alternatives. This is a good way to use up this herb when it strays out of its garden plot. You will need a 500 ml dark glass bottle and a 120 ml glass jar, both with lids.

To make the infused oil
375 ml olive oil
250 g lemon balm leaves, roughly chopped

For the wood balm
1 tbsp beeswax, grated
1 tbsp set honey
5 drops essential oil of melissa

First make the infused oil: place the oil and chopped leaves in a heatproof bowl over a pan of simmering water. Stir well so the ingredients are combined, cover and allow to simmer gently for 2–3 hours. Remove from

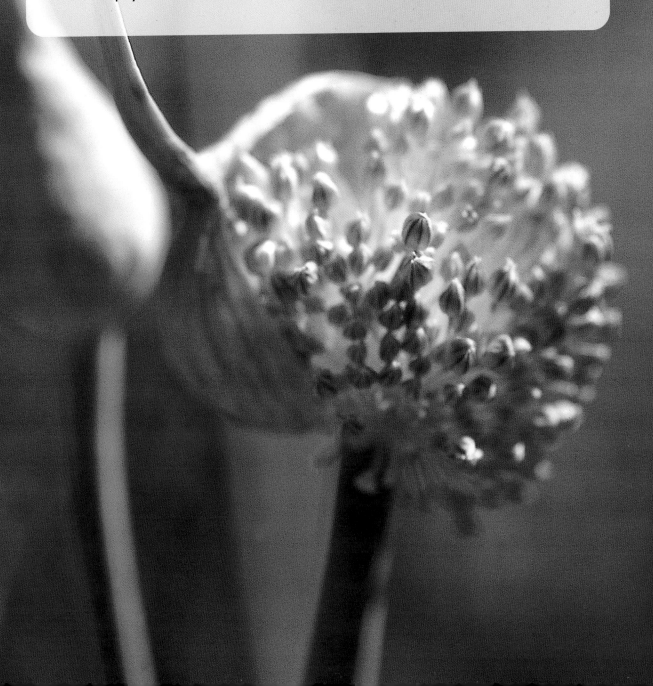

Part 3

FIRST TRIMESTER HERBS

Herbs for shock and excitement, to bolster immunity,
keep you well nourished and help you cope with nausea

Oats

calming, re-energising

The botanical name *avena* derives from the Latin *aveo*, meaning 'desire' and oats have long had a reputation as an aphrodisiac. Dreaming of oats is said to augur a long, happy partnership and a large family!

The pale gold seeds which top the stalk of the cultivated annual grass known as white oats (*Avena sativa*) support the nervous system and can lift the spirits if you are feeling stressed or anxious about your test results.

Oats raise energy levels and build stamina – perfect to counter the fatigue of early pregnancy when morning sickness can leave you feeling shattered and shaky. They can also relieve insomnia if your mind is racing more than usual at night. Oat straw – the dried stems – is the form particularly used by herbalists to support the nervous system in times of stress, for insomnia (oats are a traditional mattress stuffing) and as a tonic to increase energy and treat depression. Slow release of energy is particularly useful in the first trimester, to stave off nausea, and oats do this well. They may also help to combat cravings, especially in those trying to quit smoking.

Nutritionally, oats are rich in easily assimilated protein and a good source of soluble fibre to guard against constipation and enhance immunity. They deliver essential fatty acids, B vitamins including folate for the baby's developing nervous system and to maintain your energy reserves, and the useful minerals calcium, iron, manganese and magnesium, selenium and zinc. Applied topically, oats make a great cleanser and can soothe itchiness and dry skin.

USING THE HERB

If you feel weak or nauseous or your regular diet is disturbed by morning sickness or tiredness, reach for oats in any form – porridge, muesli, granola, cookies or flapjacks. Herbalists advise that you need 25–50 g oats daily (preferably as porridge) to counter depleted vitality, nervous exhaustion or feelings of melancholy.

To make the most of the calcium in oats – low dietary intake has been associated with an increased risk of pre-eclampsia, muscle cramps and labour pain – make porridge using 2.5 parts milk to 1 part oats. This helps to supply the extra calcium and vitamin K you need now (the latter may help to ease nausea, too). Or top a bowl of oat-based muesli or granola with yogurt. Add apricots or blueberries to sweeten with more useful pregnancy nutrients.

In cooking, substitute oats for half the flour in a crumble topping and sprinkle over gratins for extra crunchiness.

To relieve itchy or dry skin, place 6 tbsp of fine oats into a square of muslin and tie to secure. Place in the bath as you run the hot water. Use as an alternative to soap. Later on in pregnancy if your skin gets unbearably itchy, make a thick porridge of oats, allow to cool, then apply as a poultice (always see your doctor about intense itching).

For cleansing skin, pour 1 litre of boiling water over ½ cup of oats, cover and leave to cool. Strain, squeezing the porridge-like mass with the back of a wooden spoon to extract as much liquid as possible, then discard the oats. Soak cottonwool in the liquid for cleansing the face, then refrigerate until needed. Alternatively, try the skin-cleansing scrub on page 37.

To cool sunburn, relieve insect bites and other common skin complaints when travelling, soak a flannel in a decoction of oats (see oat bath recipe on page 27) and apply directly to the affected area.

To soothe tired feet at the end of the day, add a handful of oats to a footbath.

LOOKING AHEAD After the birth, ask for a bowl of caudle – a traditional food to restore energy and stamina after labour. It is made with oats, sugar, spices, honey and ale – experiment to find a taste combination you like and teach the recipe to your birth partner in advance.

OFF-THE-SHELF REMEDIES

* Choose whole organic jumbo oats, which retain their shape and bite during cooking; steel cut or pinhead oats take longer to cook. Try to avoid instant porridge mixes, which may contain additives like salt and sugar.
* Oat bran can be added to breakfast cereal, muesli and granola if the texture of porridge is a turn-off in the early weeks of pregnancy.
* If you don't have time to make flapjacks (see page 36), carry oat cakes in an airtight container in your bag for emergencies when you feel light-headed, anxious or nauseous. To turn emergency rations into an instant nutritious snack, eat with cheese and an apple.
* Look for pregnancy tonics containing oat straw if you feel exhausted, frazzled or your mind is racing.
* Oat straw tea is useful for nervous tension in pregnancy and is rated 'likely safe' by the American Pregnancy Association and the US Natural Medicines Database.

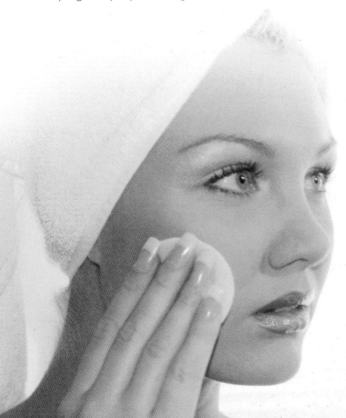

✳ Oatmilk is a good vegan substitute for soy milk during pregnancy: soy is best avoided because of the high levels of plant oestrogens it contains.

✳ Extract of oats has been shown to be useful in helping people to quit smoking; consult a herbalist for treatment before and during pregnancy.

✳ Look for oats in shampoos and conditioners for damaged hair – the hydrolysed protein in the grass is said to counter dryness and make hair look more glossy.

Nutty flapjack

The soluble fibre in oats contains beta-glucan, which slows digestion and prolongs absorption of carbohydrates into the bloodstream, keeping blood-sugar levels stable (low sugar levels can trigger nausea). As a result you're less likely to feel nauseous or exhausted. The nuts in this recipe add energising protein and omega-3 fatty acids for the baby's developing brain, eyes and nervous system.

MAKES 10–12.

125 g organic butter, plus extra for greasing
100 g muscovado sugar
2 tbsp honey
200 g organic jumbo oats
50 g walnuts, chopped
50 g dried apricots, chopped

Preheat the oven to 180°C/350°F and grease an 18 cm square shallow baking tin.

Melt the butter and the sugar in a large saucepan over a medium heat, stirring in the honey once the sugar has dissolved. Remove from the heat and stir in the oats, nuts and chopped apricots.

Tip the mixture on to the prepared baking sheet, press down and smooth out to an even thickness, then bake for 15–20 minutes, until golden brown. Remove from the oven and mark into squares. Place the tin on a wire rack and allow to cool before removing the flapjack squares.

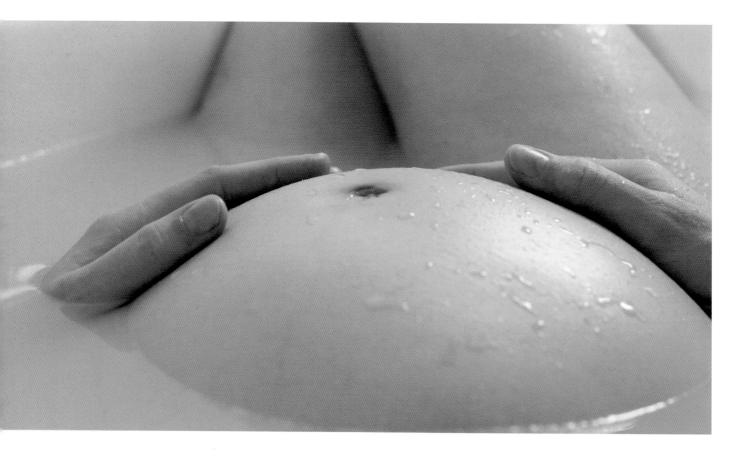

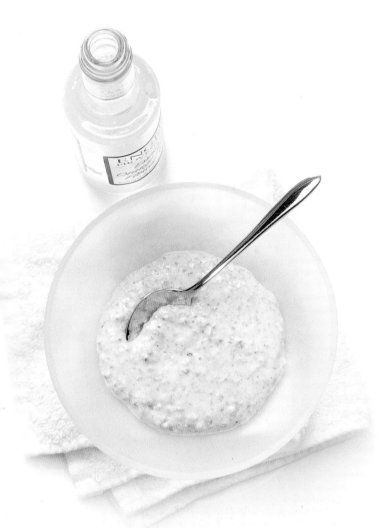

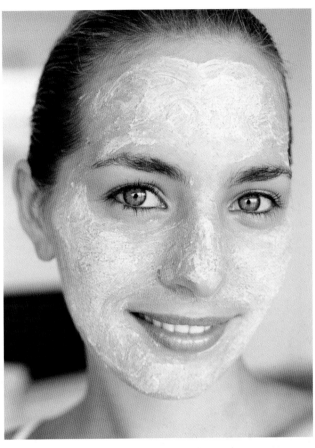

Oat bath

Making a decoction of this emollient grain helps to ease itchy skin or eczema. This bath can be particularly helpful when the skin over your belly or breasts starts to feel tight, at times of speedy growth and late in pregnancy.

40 g oats
750 ml cold water
1 tbsp grapeseed oil

Place the oats in a saucepan, cover with the water and bring to the boil. Allow to simmer for 20 minutes, uncovered, until the liquid has reduced to about 500 ml.

Strain the liquid into a jug, pressing the oats caught in the sieve with the back of a wooden spoon to extract as much of the cloudy liquid as possible. Pour the decoction into the bath and swish well to disperse. Relax in the bath for 5–10 minutes. After drying, while your skin is still damp, massage the oil into dry areas.

Oat skin-cleansing scrub

If you've decided to give up 'chemical' skincare products during pregnancy, try this gently clarifying face scrub once a week. Substitute grapeseed oil for the sweet almond oil if you are allergic to nut oils.

4 tsp fine oatmeal
4 tsp milk powder
1 tsp sweet almond oil
1–2 tbsp orange blossom water or hydrosol

Mix together the oatmeal and milk powder, then stir in the almond oil. Blend to a paste using as much orange blossom water as you need.

Massage into face and neck for a few minutes, wipe away with a warm wet flannel, then splash the skin with cool water.

Ginger

preventing nausea, soothing

In pregnancy we start to care more about the quality and purity of what we put into our bodies. In India, ginger is considered the most spiritually pure, or sattvic, of the spices; the Qur'an regards it as a holy plant.

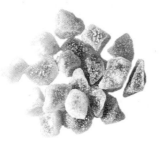

CAUTION Consult your doctor if taking blood-thinning medication, such as warfarin. Ginger root prevents blood clotting so stop using in the weeks leading up to the birth.

The rhizome of the tropical plant *Zingiber officinale* is renowned as a panacea in many of the healthcare systems of Asia, from Ayurveda in India to Jamu in Indonesia. It has been shown to be safe in pregnancy and effective at preventing and alleviating nausea – even when it has been severe. Ginger gains its remarkable powers (and zingy taste) from the phenolic compound gingerol, which also has painkilling and antibacterial properties.

The ginger rhizome works on the entire gastro-intestinal system, encouraging both appetite and digestion, countering constipation and soothing indigestion; its antiseptic properties mop up tummy bugs. The plant stimulates the circulation, making it useful if you experience cold hands and feet in late pregnancy. Its warming action promotes sweating – it can reduce a temperature and is also effective for cold symptoms since it is anti-inflammatory and a cough inhibitor.

Ginger has a soothing effect on the nervous system, and is used by herbalists to treat anxiety and depression, both of which can strike unexpectedly in the early weeks of pregnancy. Nutritionally, ginger root is a good source of minerals and vitamin B6.

CHOOSING GINGER

✳ When buying fresh ginger, look for a plump, heavy root with a sheen on the skin; avoid those that feel soft or look wrinkly. Snap off a section to check that it's juicy. There are more volatile oils in the fresh root than the dried, powdered product.

USING THE HERB

To ease pregnancy sickness, most research studies recommend 250 mg of the powdered root in capsule form, taken four times daily. Be sure to see your doctor if you don't keep down any food or drink for 24 hours or vomit after every meal.

Alternatively, keep a flask of hot ginger tea (see page 40) on your bedside table, and sip before getting up, Or have ginger biscuits or gingersnaps (see page 40) in an airtight tin next to your bed and try to nibble before first sitting up.

In Ayurvedic medicine, a combination of ginger and onions is recommended to relieve nausea and vomiting. This is also the base for most curries – try a little curry for lunch to stave off mid- to late-afternoon nausea. Or stir fry vegetables with ginger, spring onions and garlic. Sip chilled ginger ale or top up a little ginger syrup or cordial with sparkling water or any cold carbonated drink.

As a treat and to help with nausea, cut sticky crystallised ginger into small pieces to nibble on.

To relieve symptoms of colds and flu, reduce a high temperature and ease respiratory problems, drink ginger tea (see page 40). If you find the taste too hot or spicy, allow it to cool and mix half and half with mango juice, an Indian favourite. A ginger steam inhalation can also relieve cold symptoms: grate 1–2 cm of fresh root into a basin, pour over boiling water, cover your head with a towel and inhale the steam.

To soothe your stomach in the morning, try eating sweet ginger preserves with butter on wholemeal toast.

For a morning pick-me-up, add a couple of slices of fresh ginger when juicing carrots or apples. Grated fresh ginger also works well with carrot and/or apple in homemade coleslaws.

In cooking, pick off the sprouts from the eyes of ginger rhizomes and add to salads and stir-fries. Add 1–3 tsp of grated fresh ginger root to cookie doughs, cake mixtures and rice puddings. Ginger and maple syrup is a great taste combination for homemade custards and ice-creams. For a constant supply of ginger, freeze sections of fresh ginger root – it is easy to grate from frozen. Ginger graters that cut through the fibrous flesh are widely available.

LOOKING AHEAD Later in pregnancy if you feel uncomfortably 'full' or have poor peripheral circulation and suffer with leg cramps or cold hands and feet, sip ginger tea (see page 40).

After the birth, a traditional Tamil remedy for strength and healing is ginger with garlic and pepper, sweetened with jaggery (unrefined cane sugar) or palm sugar.

GROW YOUR OWN

Track ginger down in nurseries specialising in tropical plants and cultivate as a houseplant. If you have a hot, moist climate and long growing season, you can grow ginger outdoors. In spring choose fresh rhizomes with eyes, soak overnight, then plant in rich, moist, free-draining soil 5–10 cm deep, eyes facing upward. Harvest the roots after the leaves have died.

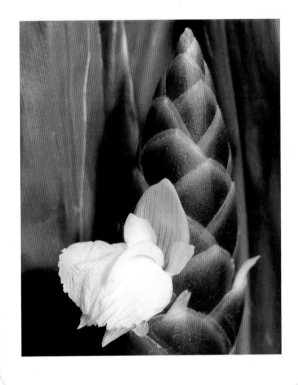

OFF-THE-SHELF REMEDIES

* Ginger tablets for travel sickness are available at health-food stores and pharmacies. Check the packet instructions for dosages during pregnancy.
* Ginger syrup, available in Asian stores, can be stirred into a cup of tea or poured over ice-cream to combat pregnancy sickness.
* Dark chocolate contains iron and potassium, both especially useful in pregnancy – bars containing candied ginger are useful treats during this trimester.

Fresh ginger tea

Take sips of this tea little and often – rather than gulping down a whole mugful – to relieve nausea. This warming tea is also comforting if you have a cold and provides a zingy wake-up call for mid-afternoon slumps, especially if you add lemon.

15 g fresh ginger root
750 ml water
honey, to taste
½ lemon, optional

Peel the ginger root, then grate into a saucepan. Add the water and bring to the boil. Allow to simmer for 15 minutes, then strain into a jug.

Pour one cup and sweeten with honey, to taste. Add a squeeze of fresh lemon juice for piquancy, if you like – the refreshing scent seems to help combat nausea, too. Store the rest of the tea in the refrigerator for up to 24 hours. Sip up to 3 cups a day.

Gingersnaps

These Scandinavian-style cookies have a satisying snap – many pregnant women find themselves drawn to crunchy textures. Older children will love helping and might like to decorate the biscuits with icing.

MAKES ABOUT 25 COOKIES

150 g organic butter, plus extra for greasing
125 g caster sugar
75 g muscovado sugar
1 egg, beaten
zest from 1 organic orange
500 g plain flour, plus extra for dusting
1 tsp baking powder
1 tbsp ground ginger
whole milk, to soften

Preheat the oven to 180°C/350°F and grease one large or two small baking sheets.

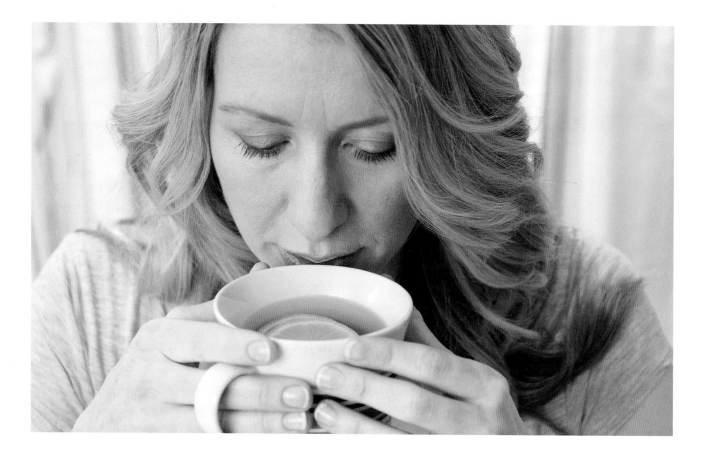

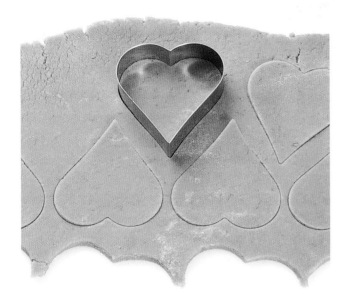

Heat the butter and sugars in a large saucepan over a medium heat. Once they have combined well and the sugar has melted, remove from the heat and allow to cool a little. Stir in the egg and orange zest, then sieve in the flour, baking powder and ginger and stir until you have a smooth dough. Loosen with a little milk, if necessary.

Roll out the dough on a floured board – the thinner you roll, the crispier the biscuits will be. Cut out shapes with biscuit cutters – hearts are traditional.

Place the cookies on the prepared baking sheet(s), and bake in batches for 10–15 minutes each, until just golden. Remove from the oven and allow to cool slightly and harden before transferring to a wire rack to cool. Once completely cool, store in an airtight container.

Ginger-infused honey

This is one of the oldest ways of preparing ginger for therapeutic use, said to date from the 6th century. Using local, unpasteurised honey makes this preparation a useful tonic if you suffer from hayfever. Drizzle over yogurt or ice-cream, use to sweeten tea or dilute with sparkling water to make a refreshing fizzy drink. You will need a 120 ml sterilised glass jar with a lid.

2 tbsp ginger root, freshly peeled and grated
6 tbsp local honey

Crush the ginger using a pestle and mortar, breaking down the fibres well. Drop the honey into the glass jar, then stir in the ginger. Make sure all the ginger is well covered by the honey. Put on the lid and refrigerate. Allow to infuse for four days before use. Use within two weeks.

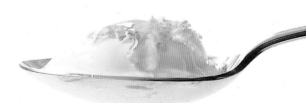

Chickpea

nourishing, beautifying

On the Greek island of Chios, a plate of chickpeas is the traditional gift brought to the home of a new mother and baby.

Nutritionally, the legume *Cicer arietinum* is an excellent choice during pregnancy. It provides good amounts of protein, making it a staple food if you are a vegetarian, and enough fibre to prevent constipation and keep blood-sugar levels stable. Chickpeas also supply folate, vital in the pre-conception period and during the first 12 weeks of pregnancy, and the minerals iron, for the manufacture of red blood cells, and phosphorus, copper and manganese for building strong bones and providing energy. In Ayurvedic medicine, chickpeas are valued for supporting growth and building up the body and are also recommended for digestive health.

Canning reduces the folate content of chickpeas by up to 45 per cent, so it's best to rehydrate then cook dried ones.

Chickpeas are particularly useful early in pregnancy if you have decided to remove 'chemical' products from your skincare regime, and if your skin has become super-sensitive. Gram flour, or besan, ground from split dried chickpeas, is one of the best-kept secrets of the Indian beauty world, where it is recommended as a gentle cleanser (or an alternative to soap) and to soothe irritated or inflamed skin. Chickpea-flour products not only leave skin feeling soft and looking less blotchy, they have useful antibacterial and antifungal properties, too. Chickpeas make such a good cleanser because they contain natural saponins – which, like soap, become foamy in water. Antioxidant saponins also seem to support the immune system, which is compromised during pregnancy.

USING THE HERB

For an energising lunchtime snack, eat falafel or hummus; both have a base of puréed chickpeas. Or make a chickpea salad (see page 44).

To blitz pregnancy pimples, make a mask by mixing a pinch of gram flour in water or natural yogurt and dab on the spot. Leave for 15 minutes then splash off with first warm, then cold, water.

For erasing dry skin on the feet, mix 1 tbsp gram flour into a paste with coconut milk and use as a scrub.

For a weekly skin scrub, add 1 tsp of crushed sesame seeds (pound them using a pestle and mortar) and a little more milk to the facial polish recipe (see opposite).

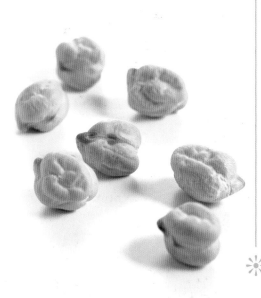

PREPARING DRIED CHICKPEAS

Dried chickpeas must be soaked before use. Place in a large bowl and cover with plenty of cold water – make sure there is at least 2.5 cm of water covering the top. Place in the refrigerator overnight. Next morning, drain the chickpeas, place in a large saucepan and cover with fresh water (don't add salt). Bring to the boil, then reduce the heat and simmer for 1½–3 hours, partially covered, until tender. Skim off scum as it rises to the surface. Drain, then the chickpeas are ready for use.

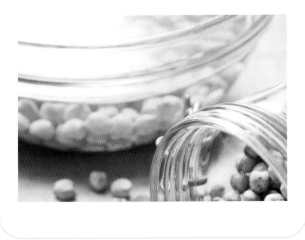

OFF-THE-SHELF REMEDIES

* Chickpea flour can be bought in South Asian stores – look for the words 'gram flour' or 'besan' on the packet.
* Sundals, snacks made from fried chickpeas, are also found In South Asian stores (if you can still tolerate – or actively crave – fried foods).

Gram flour facial polish

In India, women use this treatment to enhance the complexion, and it makes a good alternative to soap or harsh cleansing gels. You can also apply it as a mask, and use to soften the hands.

2 tsp gram flour
½ tsp olive oil
1–2 tsp whole milk

Place the flour in a small bowl and stir in the olive oil, making a thick paste. Then, little by little, stir in enough of the milk to make a smooth paste.

Apply to damp skin after removing make-up or on waking, using gentle circular movements in an upward direction and avoiding the eyes. Either splash off with warm water or, once a week, leave on as a soothing mask for 15 minutes, before rinsing off.

If you feel under the weather (as long as you have darker skin), add a pinch of turmeric powder to the facial polish recipe (see right) – this is a traditional Indian recipe for glowing good health. Avoid on light skins: it gives a yellow tinge.

As a natural hair tonic and colourant for greying hair, gram flour is used in many Indian hair and scalp treatments. Mix 2 tbsp of gram flour with water to make a paste and apply to damp hair, massaging in well. Leave for 10 minutes, then rinse out with plenty of water.

In cooking, use chickpeas whole in salads (see page 44), dahls, vegetable dishes and soups, purée for spreads and patés, and use the flour for making fritters and flat breads.The young pods and leaves of the chickpea can be eaten like spinach.

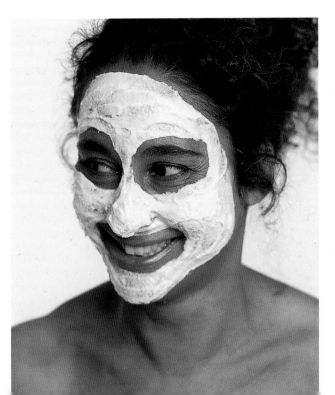

Folate-boosting chickpea salad

This couscous salad is packed with folate – not only in the chickpeas, but also in the leaves and asparagus. If asparagus is out of season, you can substitute purple-sprouting broccoli.

SERVES 2

175 g dried couscous
½ tsp dried vegetable bouillon
1 tsp orange flower water
1 tbsp extra-virgin olive oil, plus extra for drizzling
400 g cooked chickpeas
2 tbsp chopped fresh parsley
3 tbsp chopped fresh mint
juice of ½ lemon
sea salt and freshly ground black pepper, to season
100 g young spinach or beetroot leaves, roughly torn
1 bunch asparagus, woody stalks removed and steamed

Pour the couscous into a mug and note how full the mug is. Pour into a large bowl. Place the bouillon powder in the same mug and fill to the point the couscous reached with boiling water. Stir until the bouillon powder has dissolved, then pour over the couscous, stirring together well. Stir in the flower water and olive oil, and set aside for 5 minutes, covered, fluffing up with a fork occasionally.

Stir the chickpeas and herbs into the couscous, squeeze over the lemon juice and season to taste, drizzling over a little extra olive oil if necessary. Finally, add the leaves and toss to combine. Serve with the asparagus on the side.

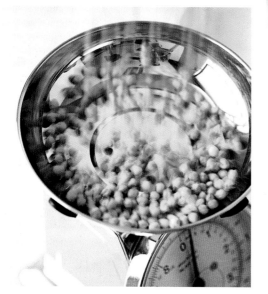

Dandelion

cleansing, supporting digestion

Blow a dandelion 'clock' or feathery seed tufts into the air calling out 'boy' then 'girl' until all the seeds have floated away. The last seed – and word – is reputed to be the sex of your baby.

A traditional tonic plant, the dandelion (*Taraxacum officinale*) can be found growing uninvited across the northern hemisphere, from lawns and roadsides to cracks in urban pavements. Its hardiness – with that deep, unshiftable taproot much maligned by gardeners – and abundance of bright flowers from early spring may have earned this plant its long associations with fecundity.

Dandelion is a bitter herb with a diuretic and laxative effect that supports the work of the liver, gallbladder and kidneys in eliminating toxins. The leaves are recommended by herbalists to combat fluid retention and the root is a mild laxative and digestive aid, relieving indigestion and bloating, and building healthy gut flora. It also stimulates the appetite. Dandelion may be prescribed to combat morning sickness.

Usefully in pregnancy, the leaves do not deplete potassium when used as a diuretic (unlike conventional medication). The herb is valued in skincare preparations for its toning action and detoxifying effect, and is used to treat acne, eczema and dry skin. Nutritionally, this plant is rich in potassium and also supplies good amounts of iron, calcium and zinc. It contains more beta-carotene than carrots, and also folate and vitamins C and D. However, dandelion should not be taken internally in large doses.

CAUTION Talk to your doctor or midwife and consult a herbalist before using if you are taking antibiotics, lithium, antacids or diuretics or medication for liver problems, or if you have high blood pressure or high blood sugar. Avoid if allergic to the daisy family.

PLANT TIPS

❋ Wear gloves when picking the plant – some people find the milky latex sap triggers an allergic rash.

❋ A dab of fresh white sap is a traditional wart remedy: warts are more common in pregnancy, when the immune system is supressed.

❋ Pick leaves for eating in spring, before the plant has flowered. Older leaves taste rather bitter. Think of dandelion leaves as wild chicory, as they do in Italy.

❋ Avoid leaves and flowers from lawns and patios, which may have been treated with weedkiller, and plants growing by busy roadsides.

❋ Harvest the root of two-year-old plants in autumn for roasting and drying.

USING THE HERB

To stimulate the appetite or ease indigestion, make dandelion leaf tea. Place 1–2 tsp of dried leaves in a teapot and pour over 250 ml boiling water; allow to steep for 5–10 minutes. Drink up to 3 cups a day. For a milder flavour use the same amount of young leaves.

For constipation and to support good bacteria in your gastrointestinal tract, make tea from the root, using ½–2 tsp dried root. Sweeten with honey if you find the brew bitter.

If you have problems digesting food, eat a few leaves before a main meal.

To cleanse oily skin, make up the dandelion cleansing milk on the opposite page.

To tone the skin or soothe sunburn, pour 1 litre of boiling water over a bowlful of flowers and leaves, cover and leave to infuse for at least an hour. Refrigerate and use as needed, dabbing on with cottonwool.

For a foot soak for puffy ankles, add a cup of dandelion vinegar (see recipe opposite) to a bowl of tepid water.

In cooking, use as an alternative to rocket or spinach in salads (see recipe opposite). Whole young leaves can be added to pizzas, steamed and added to quiches, or wilted with garlic and butter and served with a little

nutmeg. The dandelion buds, which can be sweeter tasting than the leaves, can be added to salads. Dandelion root vinegar (see recipe below) can be used to flavour salad dressings.

LOOKING AHEAD Later in pregnancy make a tincture of dandelion root (see page 13) and add to a soak for puffy ankles; this is also helpful if you suffer from constipation. Take 1–5 ml diluted in water three times daily.

If you have trouble breastfeeding, consult a practitioner of Traditional Chinese Medicine; dandelion is believed to promote lactation.

OFF-THE-SHELF REMEDIES

❋ When selecting dandelion teabags as a digestive aid, choose organic leaves in unbleached paper.

❋ Dandelion coffee – made from the roasted and ground roots – is an option if you are cutting down on regular coffee and other caffeinated drinks. Look for it in health-food stores or online.

❋ Skincare preparations make use of dandelion for its clarifying action on the skin – those from the Dr Hauschka range, grown organically, are recommended.

Dandelion root vinegar

Dandelion root adds a warm earthiness to a vinegar. Use to flavour salad dressings or top up with hot water as a drink; try sweetening with maple syrup. You will need a Kilner-style jar – the 500 ml size is good – and some clean glass bottles with lids.

handful of dandelion roots
500 ml organic cider vinegar

First get out a spade or daisy grubber and harvest a handful of roots – they look like pale carrots. Don't expect to get the whole taproot out of the ground.
Scrub the roots and remove any leaves and flowers. Dry well, then chop the roots into small chunks and place in the jar, filling it about two-thirds full.
Pour the cider vinegar over the chopped root, making sure all the root is well covered. Put the lid on tightly, then label the jar and store in a cool dark place for 4–6 weeks.
Strain through a coffee filter into the bottles, discarding the

root, and put on the lids. Label and keep in the refrigerator once opened (it will keep for up to three years in the fridge). Shake before use.

Dandelion and baby leaf salad

Including slightly bitter young dandelion leaves in springtime salads stimulates the appetite, and the lemon makes a good flavour combination. Serve with hummus and crusty bread – the thicker stems of the leaves are good for scooping.

SERVES 2

1 clove garlic, peeled
25 g young dandelion leaves, washed well
½ frisée lettuce, white inner leaves only
½ little gem lettuce
3 hard-boiled eggs, peeled and quartered
4–8 anchovies, according to taste
½ red onion, finely sliced
12 cherry tomatoes, halved
juice of ½ lemon
2–3 tbsp extra-virgin olive oil
sea salt and freshly ground black pepper, to taste

Rub the inside of a large serving bowl with the garlic clove. Cut out any thick stems from the dandelion leaves (reserve for dipping). Place the dandelion, white frisée and little gem leaves in the bowl and add the eggs, anchovies, sliced red onion and tomatoes.

In a jug whisk together the lemon juice with olive oil to taste and season. Drizzle over the salad and toss gently.

Dandelion cleansing milk

Keep this cleanser in the fridge to make the most of its refreshing properties. Make up more as you need it – it will only keep for a couple of days. It's particularly suitable for oily skin. You will need a juicer and a 500 ml sterilised glass bottle with a lid.

¼ cucumber, roughly chopped
150 ml semi-skimmed milk
15 ml dandelion tincture

Juice the cucumber and whisk the juice into the milk until well combined, then stir in the dandelion tincture. Decant into a clean bottle with a lid and refrigerate until needed. To use, shake the bottle, then apply a little of the cleansing milk to cottonwool and wipe over the face. Splash off with cool water or spritz with a flower-water hydrosol such as rose.

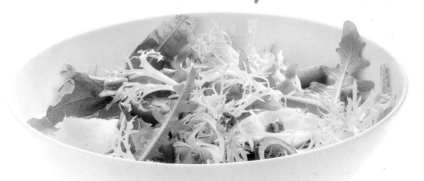

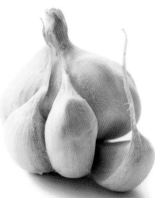

Garlic

fighting infection, improving circulation

Garlic has always been linked in folklore with babies – in many cultures the bulbs were strung up as charms to bring luck and keep evil away.

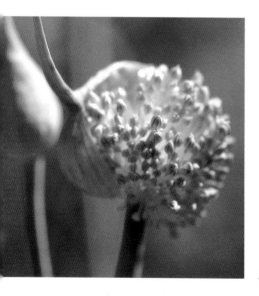

The pungent root bulb of the garlic plant (*Allium sativum*) has been used by midwives since ancient Greek times for its antibacterial and wound-healing properties, and its ability to preserve strength and endurance and bolster the body against stress and fatigue.

Garlic is antimicrobial, antiseptic, antiviral, antifungal and anti-inflammatory; it may reduce the frequency and severity of colds, clears up stomach bugs and thrush, eases chest infections, and can even overpower antibiotic-resistant bacteria like *E. coli* and MRSA. The active ingredients – organosulphur compounds including allin, allicin and ajoene – are responsible for its odour and much of the medicinal action. Alongside the antiseptic and antibiotic effects, garlic relaxes and enlarges the blood vessels, improving blood flow, and acts as an anticoagulant, which is helpful for those with varicose veins (some 40 per cent of women develop these in pregnancy). Reports suggest that garlic may be useful in pregnancy for preventing pre-eclampsia and intrauterine growth retardation.

Nutritionally, garlic is an excellent source of manganese and selenium, and also delivers calcium and phosphorus, plus vitamins B6 and C, and also boosts vitamin absorption. It seems to benefit digestion, too, encouraging the growth of good bacteria in the gut and easing bloating and wind. This is perfect for early pregnancy, when increased levels of progesterone relax the muscles in your gastrointestinal system, leading to both symptoms, at a time when you might prefer to avoid over-the-counter medications.

CAUTION Don't eat more than 2–4 cloves a day – in large quantities it is an emmenagogue – and do not eat on an empty stomach, which can bring on nausea or tummy upset. Garlic has blood-thinning properties so cut down 7–10 days before your due date to prevent excessive bleeding. Consult your doctor if you are taking anti-coagulants. Avoid if you take isoniazid, saquinavir and/or medication for HIV/AIDS.

USING THE HERB

To benefit from garlic's powers, eat 1–2 cloves of raw garlic a day. The herb's volatile oils are deactivated by cooking. Crush or cut cloves to release the active ingredients. Garlic butter is a good way to eat raw garlic – chop finely or crush and mash into butter, spread on to bread, wrap in foil and warm through in a medium oven. Alternatively, add a few crushed cloves of garlic to a bottle of olive oil, allow to steep for added flavour, and use in salads and on pizzas.

To disinfect cuts and grazes, mix up a solution of freshly crushed garlic and water.

To protect against bites if you are spending time in areas known to harbour ticks, eating garlic over a five-month period reduces the likelihood of suffering from bites. Anecdotal evidence suggests it has the same effect on mosquitoes and fleas.

As a cough remedy and decongestant, make up the garlic syrup on page 50. If eating a clove seems out of hand, crush it in a little honey to make it more palatable.

As a mouthwash, garlic can help protect delicate gums and soothe mouth ulcers (see page 50).

In cooking, garlic can be used as a flavouring in almost any type of dish. For a change, try smoked garlic bulbs – the taste combines wonderfully with a full-flavoured hard cheese. Early-harvest 'wet' garlic, available in specialist greengrocers and farmers' markets, has an especially soft and juicy flesh, a subtler flavour and deliciously wafting aroma. Chop into pasta dishes such as carbonara and grind to use in pesto (see page 50).

LOOKING AHEAD It's safe to eat garlic while breastfeeding. Although it seems to flavour breast milk, a study found that infants suckled for longer periods, sucked more and consumed more milk after their mothers started taking garlic capsules.

OFF-THE-SHELF REMEDIES

✳ If you suffer from athlete's foot, apply garlic gel containing 1 per cent ajoene – shown to be as effective as some conventional medications.
✳ Avoid processed and dried garlic products – they may be marketed as 'odourless'. They lack the health benefits of the raw cloves. A German study found that some contained no active ingredients at all.

GROW YOUR OWN

Garlic thrives over the winter, sending up fresh green shoots during the dead part of the year. It's easy to cultivate, too. Just buy the plumpest bulbs you can find in early autumn and get some pots with a diameter of at least 15 cm. Fill the pots with well-draining potting compost. Break the cloves apart and press each one about 4 cm into the compost, pointy end up (one clove per pot). Then forget about them (but water if dry) until the spring.

Harvest the green shoots from early spring; these taste milder than the bulb and make a good addition to salads, omelettes and sandwiches. The bulbs are ready to harvest when the foliage starts to yellow and die in summer.

As an alternative, in early spring look out for and pick wild garlic, or ramsons (*Allium ursinum*), from hedgerows and the verges of quiet roads or lanes. Use as you would chives, in salads and potato dishes, or grind with olive oil and sea salt into a pungent pesto using a pestle and mortar.

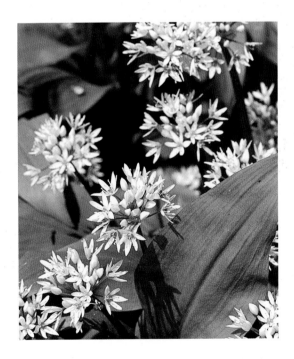

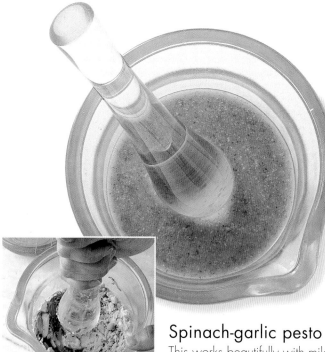

Spinach-garlic pesto

This works beautifully with mild-tasting new season garlic (when you can get away with using a little more than usual). Stir it into pasta or serve on the side with grilled fish. If you prefer less flavour or are using full-season garlic, reduce the amount to 4 cloves. If you don't have a pestle and mortar, whizz all the ingredients in a food processor.

SERVES 2

1 garlic bulb
pinch of sea salt
50 g toasted pine nuts
25 g walnuts
250 g young spinach leaves
150 g Parmesan, grated
4–6 tbsp extra-virgin olive oil

Remove the papery wrappers from the garlic cloves and crush them with the salt in a large pestle and mortar. Add the pine nuts and walnuts and crush these too, until you have an oily paste. Add the spinach leaves little by little, pounding until you have a green paste, adding a little olive oil to moisten, if necessary. Then do the same with the Parmesan and add the remaining oil until you have a green textured paste.

Garlic mouthwash

This soothes the pain of mouth ulcers and bleeding gums, which become more likely during pregnancy. In one study, a garlic mouthwash showed 'good antimicrobial activity' against streptococcus bacteria and oral micro-organisms. Results were still evident two weeks after use. Avoid if you feel extremely nauseous in this trimester.

2 cloves garlic
¼ tsp coriander seeds, optional

Peel the garlic cloves and crush into ½ a glass of tepid water. (Make sure the water is not hot or boiling, which reduces the medicinal action of the garlic.) Stir well.

Use as a mouthwash, holding the garlicky water in your mouth for as long as possible before spitting out. Repeat. If you dislike the lingering taste of the garlic, chew on the coriander seeds.

Garlic syrup

Good for coughs and colds, this cough linctus has a soothing action, thanks to the honey that preserves and sweetens the garlic. You will need two 500 ml sterilised bottles with cork stoppers. Take 1 tsp every three hours while symptoms persist.

40 g fresh garlic cloves
750 ml cold water
500 g honey

Crush the cloves (don't bother removing the papery skin) with the blade of a heavy knife and place in a saucepan with the water. Bring to the boil, then simmer until the liquid has reduced by a third which will take at least 30 minutes – you should have about 500 ml.

Strain the liquid through a sieve into another pan and add the honey. Heat gently, stirring all the time, until the honey has dissolved and the consistency is syrup-like – it should coat the back of a spoon. Remove from the heat, cover and allow to cool.

Pour the cooled syrup into the sterilised bottles using a funnel, then cork the tops. Label the bottles and store in a cool, dark place for up to six months. Shake well before use.

Part 4
SECOND TRIMESTER HERBS

Plants that aid nesting, help you get things done
and remain happy and confident

Lemon

cleansing, strengthening

Like chilli and garlic, lemon is a threshold-protection charm in India, strung or placed to repel everything from germs to ill-wishers. In the Mediterranean, its eye-like shape reputedly gives the lemon extra protective powers.

The fruit and rind of this most piquant member of the citrus family are valued for their ability to refresh, cleanse and maintain good health. *Citrus limon* has long been considered a tonic for colds, sore throats and catarrh, thanks to its antibacterial and antiseptic properties and the support it offers the immune system. And, of course, nutritionally lemons are renowned for their impressive amounts of infection-fighting vitamin C.

Lemon supports digestion: although the fruit itself is very acidic, it acts as an anti-acid and has an alkaline effect on the body, relieves gastric disorders, and is a carminative, expelling wind from the intestines. It is just the thing if your tastebuds seem to have gone haywire over the past few weeks, helping to re-establish a good appetite.

Lemon has antineuralgic properties, reducing nerve pain, and is effective as a pick-me-up, clearing the mind and reducing confusion.

The constituent bioflavonoids in lemons help to strengthen the walls of blood vessels, especially capillaries and veins, so do turn to this herb (particularly the pith and zest) if you are prone to bleeding gums or varicose veins.

The cleansing action of lemon works particularly well on the liver and pancreas, but inside the home the antibacterial and insecticidal qualities make lemon juice and oil the perfect addition to cleansing products

for safe nesting. However, the essential oil and neat lemon juice are skin irritants – the constituent bergapten, used in self-tanning products, promotes pigmentation and can sensitise the skin. Do not apply undiluted lemon juice to the skin (as a skin lightener, for example), especially before exposure to sunlight.

Vitamin C is destroyed when exposed to the air, so for the greatest health benefits, squeeze lemon juice immediately before you are going to use it.

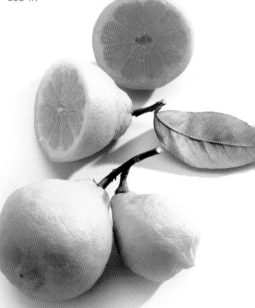

CHOOSING LEMONS

❋ Weigh lemons in your hands before buying – the finest are heavy because they are ripe with juice. They should be deep yellow and firm when pressed.

❋ Choose unwaxed organic lemons, especially when using the zest, to avoid traces of pesticides and wax treatments.

❋ Look for Italian lemons, particularly Sicilian ones raised in the volcanic soils of Mount Etna, which are perhaps the world's tastiest and juiciest. Sorrento or Amalfi lemons are also sweet enough to eat raw.

USING THE HERB

If you are still experiencing morning sickness, keep a cut lemon by your bed. Squeeze some juice into a glass and inhale before getting out of bed. Alternatively, place 2 drops of essential oil of lemon on a handkerchief and inhale.

To rouse a jaded appetite, drink a little lemon juice 20 minutes before a meal.

If your iron levels are dropping, accompany meals with a *citron pressé*: squeeze the juice of ½ a lemon into a glass and top up with hot or cold water; sweeten with a little honey. In a 1987 study, drinking lemon juice was shown to increase iron absorption. This drink is also thought to combat constipation in pregnancy.

At the first sign of a cold or fever, drink a glass of water containing the freshly squeezed juice of a lemon.

To ease sore throats, gargle with a little diluted lemon juice (mix with the same amount of water) for its astringent action. This is also effective for gingivitis and mouth ulcers.

When travelling, suck lemon sweets to keep motion sickness at bay and dab a little diluted juice on insect bites before bed.

To clean chopping boards and other kitchen surfaces, rub a chopping board with ½ a lemon. To make use of its antibacterial properties, make up a bottle of the lemon and lavender spray (see page 54) for use on surfaces.

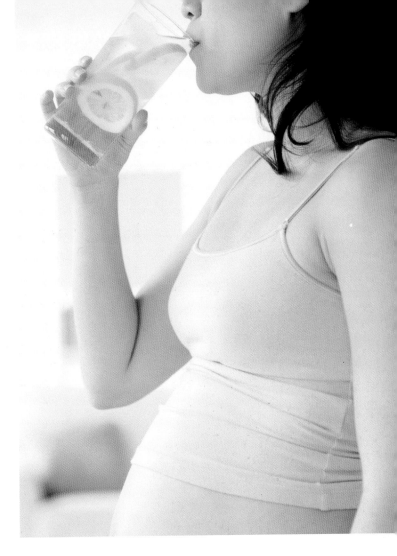

To eliminate noxious odours, place lemon quarters in bowls of water in a newly decorated room. A cut lemon will help to absorb the nauseating smells of new paint, varnish, carpets or flat-pack furniture. To keep the room smelling fresh, stud a lemon with cloves and leave in situ or create a lovely lemon garland (see page 54). A cut lemon in the fridge door will absorb lingering food smells.

To keep nails strong and stain free if you've stopped using varnish, soak them weekly in a bowl of warm water containing the juice of a lemon and ½ tsp olive oil.

To bring out blonde highlights in fair hair, use lemon juice in the final rinse water after conditioning.

In cooking, use Italian lemons sliced thinly in salads; serve drizzled with a good-quality olive oil. Add a squeeze of fresh lemon juice to shop-bought barley water as a cool-aid when you start to overheat in the second trimester or make a refreshing lemon sorbet (see page 54).

Lemon sorbet

Start or end a meal with this tart lemony delight, which is especially cooling on hot summer days as pregnancy progresses. It's a lovely treat if your growing belly makes you feel uncomfortably full at mealtimes. This is so much better for you than supermarket products since it doesn't contain artificial gums, colours or over-sweet syrups.

MAKES ABOUT 500 ML

250 g granulated sugar
250 ml water
juice of 6 lemons
zest of 2 unwaxed organic lemons

Place the sugar in a pan with the water over a medium heat and slowly bring to a simmer, stirring until all the sugar has dissolved. Then remove from the heat and stir in the lemon juice and zest (hook out and discard any pips). Allow to cool fully.

Pour into a large mixing bowl and place in an easily accessible spot in the freezer. After an hour, stir the slushy mixture with a fork or whisk, beating from the outside edge inwards to break up the ice crystals. Repeat after another couple of hours and then a third time an hour later. The beating process can take up to 5 hours. Transfer to a plastic tub and put on a lid, to freeze completely. Remove from the freezer 10 minutes before serving to allow the sorbet to soften enough to scoop. Eat within a week.

Lemon and lavender surface spray

Lemon oil has been shown to be so strongly bactericidal and antiviral that it is used in some hospitals as a disinfectant. In studies it has even been shown to wipe out airborne pathogens. This surface cleanser uses these same properties to keep the home lemon fresh. You will need a 300 ml pump-action spray bottle.

2 tsp liquid castille soap
freshly squeezed juice of 1 lemon
2 tbsp white wine vinegar
2 drops essential oil of lemon
2 drops essential oil of lavender

Put all the ingredients in the pump-action bottle and top up with at least a mug of hot water. Shake well. Wearing gloves, spray on to a surface and wipe away with a clean damp sponge or cloth.

Dried lemon garland

This is a lovely way to scent and adorn a newly decorated nursery. Dried lemon zest has long been valued as an insect repellent as well as for its refreshing piquancy.

2–3 lemons
15–20 fresh bay leaves
1 m raffia and darning needle

Preheat the oven to 150°C/300°F. Slice the lemons into 5 mm wide slices (discard the end slices) and place them on baking sheets. Make sure the slices are not touching. Place the baking sheets in the oven for at least 6 hours, or preferably overnight. Remove once the slices are dry to the touch (they should feel neither sticky nor brittle). Leave to cool.

Thread the needle with the raffia and tie a knot at the end. Thread on a lemon slice followed by a bay leaf then tie a knot. Leave a small gap and repeat. Do the same until you have used up all the dried lemon slices and bay leaves. Hang in an airy place until the bay leaves have dried out.

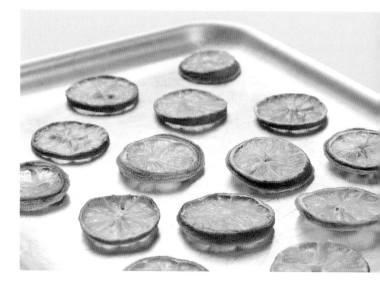

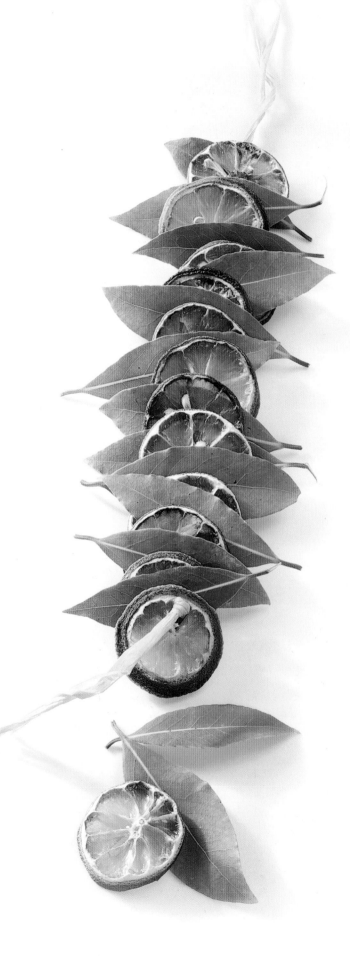

GROW YOUR OWN

A lemon tree looks – and smells – especially uplifting in midwinter, when it bears most fruit. As an added incentive to raise your own lemon tree, the pretty pink-tinged white blossom is strongly scented, as are the glossy leaves. In cooler climates choose a compact, slow-growing variety like 'La Valette' and grow it in a large container indoors or under glass. Use ericaceous compost and make sure the drainage is good; feed through the winter months with an organic fertiliser, give it a good soak regularly, and top dress yearly, replacing some of the top layer of soil with compost. Prune out dead wood or broken branches and thin twiggy growth when there is least fruit on the tree.

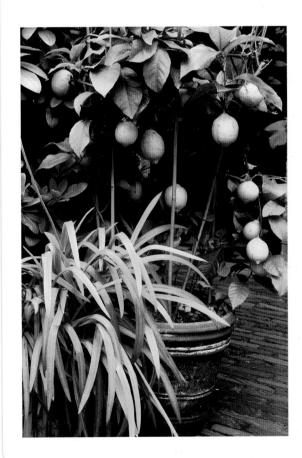

Chamomile

soothing tension, restoring calmness

The name *Matricaria* derives from the Latin *matrix*, meaning 'motherly' or 'womb-like'.

The fresh or dried flowerheads of German chamomile (*Matricaria recutita*) have a calming effect on the nervous and digestive systems and skin. If pregnancy anxieties are making you feel tense, nervous or even nauseated, this is the herb for you. It reduces irritability and promotes sleep, while easing tense or cramped muscles. Its soothing effect on the gastrointestinal organs means it can reduce wind and bloating while stimulating a jaded appetite – useful if you are beginning to get over morning sickness. Applied to the skin, chamomile can relieve the itching that can accompany a growing belly. Roman chamomile (*Anthemis nobilis*) has similar properties.

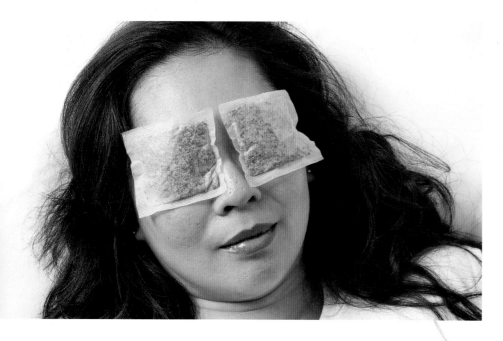

PLANT TIPS

* Pick the flowerheads in mid- to late summer on the morning of the day they open – the active ingredients are at their most potent then.
* Only pick flowers you have planted yourself so you can be sure they are the right botanical species and have been grown without harmful chemicals.
* Wear gloves when harvesting fresh flowers.

USING THE HERB

For a relaxing bedtime, make a cup of chamomile tea or use a chamomile-filled eye pillow (see page 58).

When life feels overwhelming, place 4 tsp of dried flowerheads in a jug, pour over boiling water and steep for 5 minutes before straining into a bath. The flowers look cheerful so for a quick pick-me-up, place a bunch in a rustic vase.

To ease heartburn, sip a cup of chamomile tea (see page 58) with your evening meal; its antispasmodic properties help to relieve symptoms.

If your eyes are dry or puffy, or you have dark circles due to interrupted sleep, refrigerate steeped chamomile teabags until chilled. Place one over each eye and relax for 15 minutes.

To calm itchy skin, apply steeped, cooled chamomile teabags directly to the affected area or make a pot of tea and soak a flannel in it – squeeze the cloth out and place over the skin.

For use as an all-natural rinse for light-coloured hair, see page 58.

LOOKING AHEAD Once you are breastfeeding, if your baby is windy or has colic, drink up to 3 cups of chamomile tea a day. If your baby has nappy rash, use German chamomile hydrosol to cleanse the area (after about four weeks), and add 1 tsp to his or her bathwater.

CAUTION If you are allergic to ragweed and plants in the daisy family, you may be allergic to chamomile too. Avoid if you are taking blood-thinning medication, statins or sedatives.

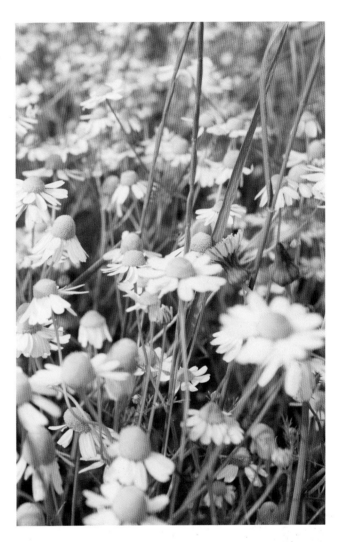

OFF-THE-SHELF REMEDIES

❋ Choose teas made from European Pharmacopoeia grade herbs, which are of higher quality than teas made from standard food-grade herbs and the interior grade herbs used in cosmetics. Brands to look out for include Traditional Medicinals and Dr Stuart's.

❋ Use a Roman chamomile hydrosol to spray insect bites or itchy skin.

❋ Homeopathic remedy Chamomilla is prescribed for toothache in pregnancy and for feelings of being unable to cope in labour. Take 6c potency.

❋ Aromatic eye pillows can be bought online from yoga suppliers, or make your own (see page 58).

❋ Chamomile creams can speed wound healing.

CHAMOMILE LAWN

A mossy, feathery chamomile lawn has been a favourite since Elizabethan times as crushed, low-growing creeping chamomile releases a grassy, apple-like scent. The herb can also be planted to create a scented path or seat, or between patio slabs. Once established, it requires only the occasional clip, though any weeds which encroach do have to be removed by hand. It also has the advantage that, unlike grass, it remains green in even the driest of summers.

Plant plugs of dense, non-flowering dwarf Roman chamomile (*Chamaemelum nobile 'Treneague'*) 15 cm apart in free-draining soil. Keep well-weeded until they spread and meld together. Don't tread on the lawn for at least three months and keep foot traffic to a minimum for the first year.

For larger areas, buy chamomile lawn as turfs.

Relaxing chamomile tea

Sipping a cup of freshly brewed chamomile tea before bed should soothe the nerves and ease heartburn that worsens at night. This herb is high in calcium and magnesium, which you need more of during pregnancy. Do not drink more than 1 cup; the herb has long been used as an emmenagogue, stimulating blood flow in the uterus and pelvis.

1 tsp dried chamomile (*Matricaria recutita*) flowers
1 mug freshly boiled water
honey or lemon, to taste

Place the flowers in a warmed teapot and pour over the boiled water. Allow to steep for 3 minutes then strain into a cup. Sweeten with honey or make more refreshing with a squeeze of lemon. Drink hot.

Chamomile hair rinse

The golden flowers of chamomile famously lighten blond and red tones and refresh highlights without the need for chemicals; this also brings a sparkle and softness to dry hair. The steam feels good if you have a cold.

25 g dried chamomile (*Chamaemeles nobile*) flowers
500 ml boiling water

Place the flowers in a teapot or ceramic jug with a lid. Pour over the water, put on the lid or cover and allow to stand for 20 minutes.

Strain the warm chamomile infusion into a jug. Shampoo and condition your hair as normal, then towel dry. Pour the chamomile infusion over your hair, catching it in another bowl and repeating the rinse 6 time sor more.

Wrap your head in an old dark towel for 20 minutes (the infusion will stain a pale towel) then rinse with warm, then cold water. Dry and style as usual.

Calming chamomile eye pillow

To bring on sleep, call on the sedative properties of chamomile; this herb is also a traditional nightmare remedy, worth trying if thoughts of change and labour are preying on your mind. The linseed in the pillow adds a weight that feels comforting if you have a headache.

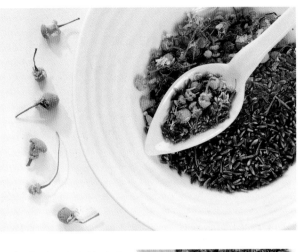

25 x 25 cm piece of cotton lawn or flannel
1 tbsp dried chamomile (*Matricaria recutita*) flowers
1 tbsp dried lavender flowers
250 g linseed *(flaxseed)*
1m silk ribbon, 2 cm wide, optional

Fold the fabric in half (right side together) to produce a rectangle measuring 25 x 12.5 cm. Lleaving a seam of at least 1 cm, sew three edges together: stitch along one of the shorter edges, the long edge and half of the other shorter edge, leaving a gap at the end. Turn the fabric case inside out, pushing the corners out with the tip of a pair of scissors or seam ripper. Press flat with an iron. Add

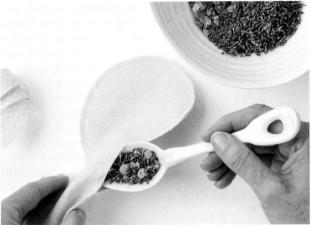

the chamomile and lavender flowers to the case then enough linseed to fill the case three-quarters full. Sew up the remaining short side of the case.

To use, shake the pillow so the seeds are in the centre and place over your eyes and sinus area. Make sure the bag cuts out the light, then drift off, focusing on the scent.

You can warm the bag in a microwave (check after 20 seconds) to boost its aromatic properties, or chill in the refrigerator and place at the base of your neck to relieve a pregnancy headache.

For a professional look, create a basic mask template and use this to cut out two mask-shaped pieces of fabric. Stitch the two pieces together, right sides out, leaving a gap at one end. Fill and stitch the gap closed. Trim the seam slightly, then finish by covering with the ribbon.

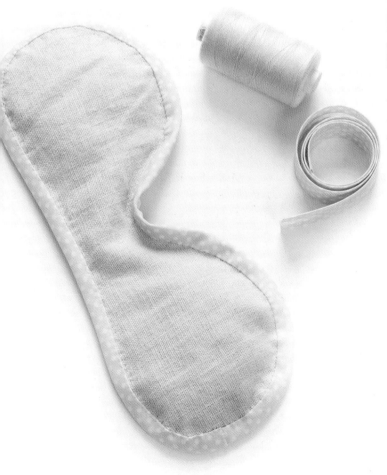

Blueberries

preventing infection, building good health

Native Americans regarded the five-pointed star-end of a blueberry as an auspicious sign. Many plants associated with women's reproductive health share this symbolic pentagram.

Native to North America, these sweet berries from the genus Vaccinium have the highest antioxidant capacity of any fresh fruit, thanks to the constituent phenolic compounds called anthocyanins, which also give them their anti-inflammatory, anti-blood clotting and antibacterial properties.

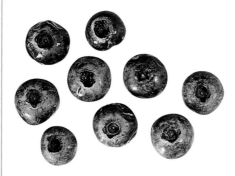

Many health studies have been conducted on the *Vaccinium corymbosum*, the highbush and most widely cultivated commercially blueberry. The more scrubby lowbush type (*V. angustifolium*) is the wild species which is also raised commercially. If you get the choice, choose *V. angustifolium*, which contains greater amounts of antioxidants. The riper the berry, the more antioxidants – studies suggest blueberries have more of these than kale, broccoli, strawberries and spinach.

Darker fleshed European bilberries (*V. myrtillus*) also have these antioxidant effects and are thought to contain more phenolic compounds

than North American blueberries (525 mg per 100 g compared to 325 mg). Bilberries taste a little more acidic than blueberries, so are more widely available in compotes, jams and jellies, rather than as fresh fruits.

Eating a large handful of fresh berries (about 30) daily helps in the formation of connective tissue, and strengthens and relaxes blood vessels, regulating blood pressure. This can be beneficial for those suffering from varicose veins, poor circulation and haemorrhoids. Other constituents – ellagic acid and pectin – are beneficial for the gastrointestinal system, while tannins act on the urinary tract in a way similar to cranberries (*V. macrocarpon*), to prevent infection. Studies on older people have linked consumption of blueberries with short-term memory enhancement.

Nutritionally, these berries are packed with vitamins C, B, E and K, manganese and have one of the highest concentrations of iron of a temperate fruit. In a study reported in the journal *Epidemiology*, pregnant

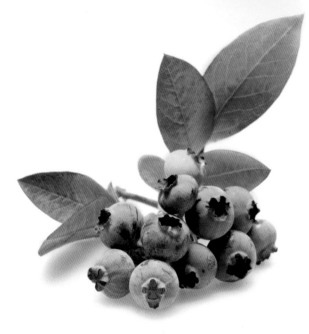

For bleeding gums and mouth ulcers, juice some berries, dilute with a little water, then use as a mouthwash. Do swallow to make the most of the antiseptic and anti-inflammatory properties.

If you have diarrhoea, the dried berries have a binding action, and are said to be an effective remedy. Chew on a handful or crush 20 g and simmer in 750 ml water for 20–30 minutes to make 3–4 cups. Drink through the day, as necessary.

OFF-THE-SHELF REMEDIES

❋ Out of season, dried berries make a chewy treat and good alternative for raisins in cooking – you need fewer of these daily, approximately 20–60 g.

❋ Frozen blueberries are a good alternative to fresh; they retain their phytonutrients (which are lost in other processing methods).

❋ When choosing berry teas or infusions, look for mixes containing bilberries, cranberries, blackberries and blackcurrants. Some come blended with black tea if you prefer a more astringent cup that tastes less like fruit punch.

women who ate vitamin-C-rich foods were shown to have a lower risk of pre-eclampsia. Blueberries contain fibre, too, to prevent constipation.

USING THE HERB

Eat out of hand Berries eaten without cooking – straight from the carton or bush (look for pick-your-own farms specialising in soft fruit from mid-summer) – will ensure you get the most of the vitamin C and anthocyanins (the latter cluster in the skin) they contain. Processed berries – for example, in compotes, yogurts and juices – don't have the same potency. Start the day with a handful of berries on muesli, pancakes, yogurt or porridge.

In cooking, Try the delicious smoothie and muffins on page 62. A blueberry sauce or coulis is easy to make and delicious over ice-cream.

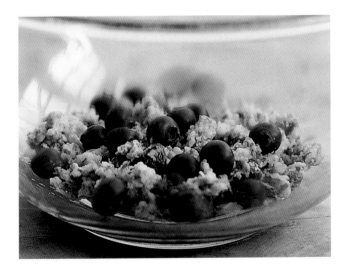

GROW YOUR OWN

Blueberries can be container grown and are more resistant to pests than many other fruiting plants. They also look attractive in early spring with their masses of waxy white flowers. Choose a large pot and acidic ericaceous compost, which needs to be kept moist, and site in a sunny position, sheltered from strong winds. Every winter prune away dead or non-fruiting branches (these are darker in colour) and in early spring scrape away a good layer of soil from the top of the pot and add a new layer of ericaceous compost. The berries are ready to harvest from mid-summer into autumn, when dark indigo and firm, with a shimmery silver bloom.

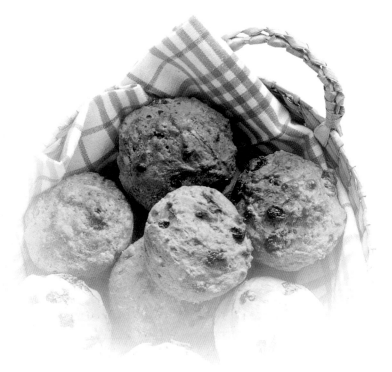

Calcium-rich berry smoothie

These berries are great for the veins and for supporting the immune system. The yogurt in the mixture contributes much-needed calcium and the ripe banana adds sweetness.

100 g natural yogurt
100 g fresh or frozen blueberries
6 strawberries
½ ripe banana, sliced

Place all the ingredients in a blender and pulse until smooth. Add a little water if you find the consistency too stiff, and blend again. Serve over ice if pregnancy is making you superhot or if (like many pregnant women) you simply crave the crunch of ice.

Blueberry muffins

The Iroquois people of North America were the first known to add blueberries to muffin mixtures. The cornmeal adds a welcome crunchy texture at breakfast time. These muffins aren't over-sweet, but are full of gooey berries.

MAKES 12

100 g organic butter, brought to room temperature
50 g soft brown sugar
2 eggs, beaten
75 g self-raising flour
25 g fine polenta (cornmeal)
125 g fresh blueberries

Preheat the oven to 200°C/400°F, and line a deep, 12-hole regular (not mini) muffin tin with paper muffin cases.

Cream together the butter and sugar until you have a light, fluffy mixture. Add the beaten egg little by little, sifting over a little flour and stirring between each addition to prevent curdling. Sift over and mix in the remaining flour, then fold in the polenta and the berries.

Divide the mixture between the cases. Bake for 15–20 minutes, until risen and golden on top. Transfer to a wire rack to cool. Serve warm or cold.

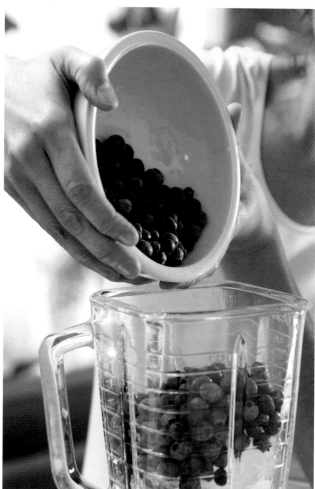

Apples

nourishing and supporting good health

Apples were a symbol of Pomona, the Roman mother goddess, who represented completion and fruition – bringing things successfully to term.

'Bloom well and bear well' is a traditional English wassailing greeting to an orchard of apple trees each winter to ensure fertility. This tree of life (*Malus domestica*) has long been a symbol of swelling hope and constant renewal; it remains 'gracious' and 'noble' (according to the 13th-century scholar and theologian Bartholomeus Anglicus) despite assault by the forces of nature. Early medical writers recommended apples to counter depression – Robert Burton describes them in his *Anatomy of Melancholy* of 1621 as 'good against melancholy' and John Caius, physician to Queen Elizabeth I, held that the scent alone would help those feeling under the weather to recover strength.

The antioxidant flavonoids in apples strengthen our health. These cluster in and around apple skin so always eat the skin as well as the flesh (but make sure apples are thoroughly washed).

Apples contain some of the highest levels of the phenolic compound quercetin, which has an anti-inflammatory action, prevents blood cells from clumping together and regulates blood pressure; another flavonoid, phlorizin, supports the lungs. One research study has suggested that mothers who ate apples during pregnancy could reduce their child's risk of developing asthma. Easy to digest, apples contain malic and tartaric acids which reduce acidity and inhibit fermentation in the intestines. The soluble fibre pectin also encourages beneficial gut flora to flourish while balancing blood-sugar levels. Nutritionally, apples provide vitamin C, folate, potassium and lots of fibre to prevent pregnancy constipation – just one apple can provide 15 per cent of your daily fibre requirements.

CHOOSING APPLES

❋ To check whether an apple on a tree is ready for picking, cup it in the palm of your hand and push upwards. If it comes free easily, it's ready; if not, try again in a few days.

❋ Don't worry about how old your apples are: one study has shown that even after 200 days, apples retained almost as many flavonoids as those which had been freshly picked.

❋ Buy organic to avoid ingesting wax and pesticide residues on the all-important skin. A study at the Swiss Research Institute of Organic Agriculture found that organic apples have higher levels of phenolic compounds than conventionally grown apples.

❋ Red apples are a better source of the beneficial flavonoid quercetin, a powerful antioxidant.

❋ Cooking apples are more acidic, larger in size, and have more flavour and 'bite' than dessert apples. The more acidic the apple, the quicker it breaks down into a purée, and so the better for baking. At the start of the season, 'cookers' have more acidity; towards the end of the season they may become more dessert-like.

❋ Dessert varieties contain more sugar than cooking varieties and are sweeter in flavour. Some need careful storage to develop their mature flavour.

USING THE HERB

To ease a dry cough, try the traditional remedy of steamed apples sweetened with honey to encourage mucus from the lungs.

For a sore throat, mix 2 tsp of apple cider vinegar in a mug of water and use as a gargle.

As an aid to digestion, serve apples with rich foods such as pork and goose, and cheese. The ancient Greeks considered an apple a good way to end a meal.

To massage sore gums, eat a raw apple; this is also an old tooth-cleaning remedy.

For bowel problems, grated apple is a German remedy for diarrhoea while stewed apple can relieve constipation.

To remove built-up hair product and add shine, after washing and conditioning your hair, add 1 cup of apple cider vinegar to the final rinse water.

OFF-THE-SHELF REMEDIES

❋ Choose cloudy over clear apple juice. Research has found cloudy apple juice to be more beneficial for the heart and lungs than regular apple juice.

❋ Apple cider vinegar, made by leaving cider to 'rest' in wooden barrels, is thought to help indigestion; use it in salad dressings. Don't worry about the alcohol; the fermentation process turns it into acetic acid.

❋ The Bach Flower Remedy Crab Apple© (*Malus sylvestris* is the wild version of the tree) is recommended if you are concerned about your new shape – it nurtures confidence and pride in the beauty of your bump, and helps morning sickness, too. This 'cleansing' remedy is useful if you find yourself obsessing over minutiae or worrying about having to have everything clean before the baby arrives, simply put 2 drops in a glass of water and sip as required until symptoms subside.

Cider vinegar toner

The natural acidity in this fermented vinegar helps to regulate the pH (alkalinity or acidity) of the skin. The orange flower hydrosol adds a feminine scent and suits dry or sensitive skin. You will need two 100 ml clean bottles with lids.

100 ml cider vinegar
100 ml orange flower water or hydrosol

Simply pour the vinegar and flower water in equal quantities into the clean bottles. Put on the lid tightly and shake well to combine. Label and store in a cool, dark place. To use, soak cottonwool with the toner and wipe over a clean face, avoiding the eye area.

Apple face mask

The original 'pomade' or pomatum – an ointment for rough skin made from apple pulp, lard and rosewater – takes its name from the Latin word for apple. The malic acid in apples is a natural alpha-hydroxy acid, which removes dead cells from the surface when applied to the skin, speeding up skin renewal. This mask can be useful for softening skin, making it look noticeably fresher. If you have oily skin, just apply grated apple. You can buy the dried clay from health stores or online.

½ apple, cored
2 tbsp runny honey
2½ tbsp bentonite clay

Grate the apple into a ceramic or glass bowl and add the honey and dried clay, mixing until you have a sticky paste.

Apply to a dry, cleansed face, avoiding the eye and mouth areas, and relax for 10–15 minutes. Try not to move or it might slide off! Splash off the mask with cool water.

Wassail bowl

This is a warming winter drink to share, traditionally served on Twelfth Night during the wassailing, or blessing, of an orchard. It's usually made from cider (though this version is non-alcoholic) and served in a large wooden vessel with a slice of toasted brown bread floating on the top. Experiment with this if you wish.

MAKES 1 LITRE

1 litre cloudy apple juice
1 stick cinnamon
4 cloves
1cm fresh ginger root, sliced
zest and juice of 1 lemon, pips removed
1 organic apple, cored and sliced
1 organic orange, halved and sliced, pips removed
2 tbsp honey
freshly grated nutmeg

Place all the ingredients in a large saucepan over a medium heat and bring to the boil. Reduce the heat and simmer for 10 minutes. Serve warm.

Seaweed

boosting immunity, cleansing

In Japan they say that eating seaweed during pregnancy ensures that your baby will have beautifully thick, glossy hair. Thanks to its root-like holdfast that clings to a rock, seaweed is also a symbol of steadfastness.

The fresh and dried fronds of many sea plants contain polysaccharides (a form of soluble fibre) that are soothing for the digestive system, and recommended if you suffer from indigestion or have vomited a lot through the first trimester.

The sodium alginate present in seaweeds forms a thick gel when it comes into contact with water. In the body it can bind with toxins, making it ideal for speeding their passage through the digestive system. The most effective seaweeds for this are kelp and bladderwrack (*Fucus vesiculosus*). In Traditional Chinese Medicine and Ayurvedic medicine, brown kombu kelp (*Saccharina latissima*) is considered a 'salty' taste and is prescribed to promote urination and to treat oedema.

Seaweed's cleansing ability makes it an effective beauty aid, as do its smoothing and firming properties. These produce an antiweathering effect, while the iodine they contain helps to repair sun damage. The high mineral content gives the effect of a mini-lift when seaweed is applied to the skin, and its nutrients stimulate the collagen-producing cells for a skin-plumping effect. Herbalists use seaweed to boost energy levels, combat stress and fatigue, and support the immune system.

Nutritionally, seaweed is one of the richest plant sources of vitamins and minerals, containing impressive amounts of B vitamins including folate and beta-carotene, and vitamins C, E and K. The minerals include large amounts of iodine, needed to balance the thyroid gland which works harder in pregnancy, as well

CAUTION Avoid all seaweed if you are allergic to iodine. Avoid kelp if you are taking antithyroid, anticoagulant or antiplatelet medication. Kelp slows blood clotthing so stop use in the weeks leading up to the birth. Avoid seaweed wraps in spas and salons; during pregnancy, these can be too heating and dehydrating.

as selenium, zinc, copper and manganese, plus calcium, magnesium and fluorine for healthy teeth and bones.

PLANT TIPS

❋ Harvest fresh, live seaweed in spring and early summer (autumn is the best season for laver). It will be fresh if rooted to a rock. Never use seaweed that has been washed up on the shore or is floating on the ocean surface. The best time to start harvesting is a couple of hours before low water. Snip off the top of the plant, leaving the root to regrow.

❋ Always use an identification guide and don't take anything you can't recognise. Most seaweed is edible, but some varieties don't taste good.

❋ Contact the water authority or environment agency to find out about water quality before picking seaweed to eat. The best places to collect are unpolluted bays that are washed daily by the tide. Avoid those near busy towns or tourist destinations.

❋ Rinse seaweed well just before cooking to remove sand and tooth-breaking grit. Don't rinse and store though – rinsing triggers the decomposition process.

USING THE HERB

For skin problems such as pregnancy acne, use a seaweed face mask (see page 68) weekly. For dry skin on your feet, try a seaweed soak (see page 68).

To ease a sore throat, particularly if coughs disturb your sleep, sip a little of the soothing throat balm (see page 68) before bed.

For low iron levels, add wakame, which is high in iron, to dishes.

In cooking, powdered kelp makes a good -substitute for salt, while laverbread can be combined with chopped bacon and oats, formed into patties and pan fried on both sides until golden brown for a breakfast treat. Use dried wakame (*Alaria esculenta*) and arame kelp in slow-cooked casseroles and rice dishes. Both are good sources of protein although arame kelp is sweeter and nuttier. Carrageen, or Irish moss (*Chondrus crispus*), is the most gelatinous seaweed; use as a nutritious setting agent in milky puddings and jellies (the flavour combines well with chocolate and vanilla). Sprinkle dried powdered nori flakes over fish dishes and salads for an extra-savoury tang.

OFF-THE-SHELF REMEDIES

❋ E numbers E400 to E405 are a sign of kelp alginates in foods, used to bind or emulsify ingredients. E406, E407 and E407a indicate carrageen, the vegetarian alternative to gelatine.

❋ On skincare products, look for the word 'carrageenan' on the ingredients list; this can help soothe itchy skin.

❋ The Welsh speciality laverbread, sold in tins in delis and online, is made by boiling red Porphyra for some hours, until reduced to a dark-green, gelatinous paste.

❋ Avoid seaweed tablets or capsules: dried or fresh seaweed has more nutritional value and tastes better.

Dulse
Reddish-purple dulse (Palmaria palmata) is especially rich in potassium. This is one of the mildest tasting seaweeds.

Porphyra
Nori or laver (Porphyra) contains the greatest amounts of protein; it's the one used in sushi wraps and miso soup.

✳ Seaweed soaps have a lovely gelatinous quality and suit super-sensitive skin. Those made from wild-harvested seaweed are reliably good.

Seaweed soak

Bathwater heated to 34–37°C causes widening of the blood vessels in the skin, allowing the mineral contents of the water to penetrate the skin.

50 g dried kelp
20 cm x 20 cm muslin square
2 tbsp sea salt, finely ground
2 tbsp olive oil

Crumble the seaweed into the centre of the muslin and tie to secure. Run a bath and throw in the muslin bag.

In a large bowl, stir into the salt enough of the oil to make a medium-thick paste. Use as a foot scrub, rubbing handfuls into your heels and balls of the feet. You might also like to tackle your elbows if they too are feeling rather hard and dry.

Rinse off the salt with a warm wet flannel. Step into the bath for a 5–10 minute soak, inhaling the salty marine scents. Rub the bag over your arms and legs, hands and face, and nails to soften them.

Seaweed acne mask

If you suffer from pregnancy acne or tired skin, use this mask weekly.

1 tsp dried rose petals
2 tbsp kelp powder
2 tbsp honey
1–2 tsp rosewater or hydrosol, optional

Pound the dried petals to a powder using a pestle and mortar. Place the kelp powder in a ceramic or glass bowl and stir in the honey to make a sticky paste; thin with a little rosewater if you prefer a less gloopy consistency.

Apply a thin layer to cleansed skin, avoiding the eye and mouth areas. Lie down and relax for 10 minutes, then rinse off by splashing with first warm, then cool, water.

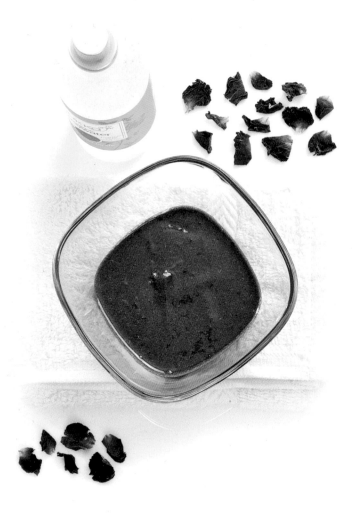

Sore throat balm

This soothing drink calls on the gelatinous properties of carrageen or Irish moss, which is softening and protective as well as being antimicrobial and antiviral.

10 g dried carrageen (*Chondrus crispus*)
750 ml water
juice of ½ organic lemon
1 tsp honey, or to taste

Soak the seaweed in water for about an hour, until nicely soft, then rinse with fresh water and place in a large saucepan with the water. Bring to the boil, reduce the heat and simmer, covered, for 30 minutes, or until the consistency is jelly-like. Pour out a mugful and add the lemon juice and honey.

Place the remaining infusion in a jug and refrigerate. On cooling, it will harden; to bring back to a liquid form, reheat, and add more lemon and honey to taste.

Part 5

THIRD TRIMESTER HERBS

Plants to tone and build endurance,
encourage relaxation and ease labour

Red raspberry leaf

toning the uterus, speeding delivery

In Hawaiian mythology, the first wild raspberry vines sprang from the skirts of Haumea, the ancestress from whom all Hawaiian people are descended and whose name derives from a word meaning 'sacred birth'.

Tea made from red raspberry leaf (*Rudus idaeus*) is perhaps the best known of pregnancy herbal remedies, recommended by herbalists, natural birth advocates and many midwives to prepare the uterus for delivery – to make contractions more effective, shorten the length of labour, and reduce the risk of early or late delivery.

The leaves of red raspberry are traditionally used to improve digestive disorders. They contain tannins (which have an astringent action that can strengthen tissues) and ellagic acid (which has an antioxidant, anti-inflammatory and antibacterial effect and relaxes the blood vessels). However, the tannins in raspberry leaves may inhibit iron absorption (and also absorption of calcium and magnesium) – so wait for two hours after drinking it before eating iron-rich foods.

During the third trimester, red raspberry leaves are recommended to tone the muscles of the uterus and aid elasticity, making contractions, when they come, more effective, so that labour progresses more steadily. During labour, sipping the tea has been said to ease pain. In 1832, the American herbalist Samuel Thomson said, 'It is the best thing for women in travail of any article I know of.' After the birth, the tea is recommended for its restorative properties.

There is no evidence that red raspberry leaf induces labour. However, an Australian study in 2000 showed that mothers who took the herb daily from 32 weeks tended to have a significantly shorter second stage of labour and a lower rate of forceps intervention than those who did not. Herbalists have also used this herb to treat sore throats and stomach upsets.

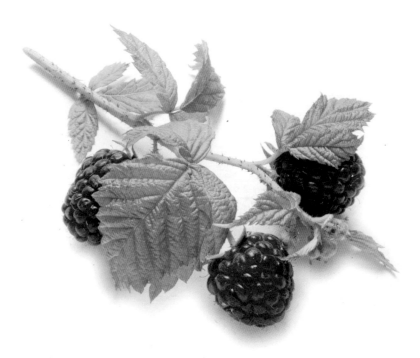

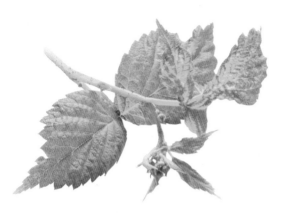

Nutritionally, it contains vitamins C and E and beta-carotene and the minerals iron, zinc and an absorbable form of calcium. Always tell your doctor and midwife when you start to take this herb.

PLANT TIPS

❋ Only pick fresh leaves if you know the cultivar of the plant. Pick young leaves (while the plant is flowering) and avoid older, wilted or partly dried leaves.

❋ To dry your own leaves, arrange on trays and place on a sunny windowsill. Turn regularly until dried completely on both sides. Once fully dry, store in an airtight container in a cool, dark place.

USING THE HERB

As a uterine strengthener, the herb takes a while to have an effect. Start drinking 1 cup of tea a day from week 32, building up over the weeks to 3 cups daily.

To combat sore gums and mouth ulcers, try using the tea on page 72 as a mouthwash from 32 weeks.

To help stem diarrhoea, drink the tea cold. However, if you suffer from constipation, be aware that the tannins in the leaves could make it worse.

To treat nausea and bleeding gums earlier in pregnancy, a herbalist may prescribe the tea. If so, follow his or her prescription.

For tired eyes, and to treat minor cuts and leg ulcers, make up the wound soak infusion on page 72

To assist with labour, make up a flask of the tea, sweetened with honey or pour cooled, sweetened tea into ice cube moulds, and take the ice cubes in a freezer bag to suck during labour.

If you are overdue, drinking more tea will not bring on labour. Consult a herbalist about blends that mix this leaf with blue cohosh and squaw vine once labour has started, to speed things up.

LOOKING AHEAD To speed healing after the birth, continue drinking the tea. It has antibacterial qualities and immune-supporting nutrients, and is said to help maintain a plentiful supply of milk. It also stimulates the uterus to start returning to its pre-pregnancy condition, and may ease after-pains.

To ease the symptoms of mastitis, soak the leaves and apply as a poultice directly to the breast.

OFF-THE-SHELF REMEDIES

❋ Raspberry fruit tea is not a substitute – it does not have the same medicinal effects.

❋ Raspberry leaf in tablet form (1.2 g daily), taken from 32 weeks onwards, was reported in the Australian study to have no adverse effects for mother or baby.

❋ If you prefer to take a liquid extract – which can be less hassle in the days leading up to labour – take 4–8 ml of the 1:1 preparation three times daily.

❋ From 38 weeks onwards, look out for pregnancy teas that combine raspberry leaf with other birth-preparation herbs, such as motherwort. Do not take earlier in pregnancy.

CAUTION Avoid this herb if you have previously had speedy deliveries (less than three hours from first contractions) or are expecting a small-for-dates baby. Consult your doctor and midwife before taking if you have had a previous caesarean, premature labour or vaginal bleeding or if there is breast or ovarian cancer in the family, endometriosis or fibroids, you have blood-pressure problems or are expecting twins. Avoid if the birth is being induced.

Red raspberry leaf and lemon verbena tea

Red raspberry leaf doesn't make the sweetest tasting of teas – it's extremely astringent. A little lemon verbena in the mix adds a delicate perfume and citrus taste that makes the brew more palatable.

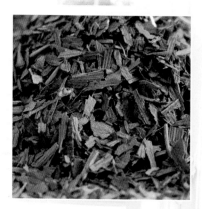

15 g dried organic red raspberry leaves
5 g dried lemon verbena leaves
500 ml just-boiled water
honey, to taste

Place the leaves in a teapot and pour over the water. Leave to steep for 10–15 minutes. Strain into a cup and sweeten to taste with the honey. To reserve the tea for later, strain into a jug and leave to cool. Once cold, put on a lid and refrigerate. Either warm up again or drink cold.

Wound soak

This cold infusion uses the astringency of the leaves to reduce inflammation and tighten the membranes surrounding a wound. The same preparation has served as an eyewash for centuries – the Irish herbalist John K'Eogh described its use back in 1735. It can be used earlier than 32 weeks.

25 g dried or 75 g fresh red raspberry leaves
500 ml just-boiled water

Place the dried or fresh leaves in a warmed pot or jug with a lid and pour over the water. Put on the lid and allow to infuse for 10 minutes. Strain and leave to cool, then store, covered, in a cool place for up to 24 hours.

To use, soak a cottonwool swab in the infusion and apply to wounds and varicose ulcers or use in an eyebath for sore eyes.

Lavender

relaxing, relieving pain

The name 'lavender' derives from the Latin *lavare*, to wash, a testament to its effectiveness in ensuring the cleanliness of delivery rooms and nurseries.

The flowers of the lavender plant (*Lavandula angustifolia*) yield a volatile oil that is simultaneously relaxing and stimulating for mind and body. The flowers are used by herbalists and the oil by aromatherapists to calm the nerves, treat mood swings and reduce muscle tension, including tension that manifests as headaches and digestive problems. Lavender has sedative properties, making it useful for treating insomnia, irritability and anxiety.

Trials have shown that inhaling lavender oil can decrease the heart rate and bring about a feeling of calm. In animal studies, lavender has been shown to reverse caffeine-induced hyperactivity – worth a try if your impending delivery date is causing masses of activity or over-excitement. Lavender also lifts the spirits and stimulates the mind, increasing mental performance, lifting exhaustion and making you feel more positive and vigorous.

One study found that after inhaling the scent, anxious people felt less fatigued, making this herb useful in the last few weeks of pregnancy when everything can seem just too much effort, physical and mental. Lavender has antibacterial, antiseptic and insecticidal properties, and has been used post-operatively to treat pain. A study of women postnatally found that they felt less discomfort between days 3–5 when they bathed with lavender; lavender baths also seem to enhance well-being and ease the blues. Other studies have shown that the scent of lavender reduces the memory of an intense and unpleasant painful experience.

CAUTION Stop using two weeks before a scheduled caesarean – its effect on the central nervous system may interfere with anaesthesia and post-surgical medication. Talk to your doctor before using if you are taking sedatives or antidepressants.

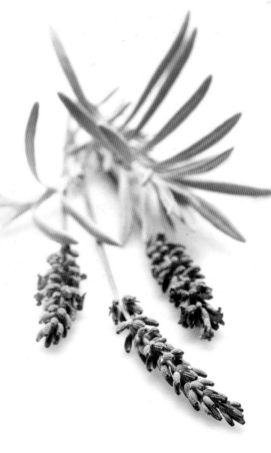

MAKING LAVENDER WANDS

Lavender wands are decorative and add a lovely scent to drawers and linen cupboards. You will need about 2 metres of narrow ribbon and at least a dozen lavender stems (an odd number works best), trimmed of leaves but with flowerheads intact. Tie the stems together just below the flowerheads, leaving one long end of ribbon. Now start to weave the long end of ribbon under and over the stems, enclosing the flowerheads in the middle. Continue working under and over the stems until you have completely enclosed the flowerheads and reached the end of the stems, then tie off the ribbon.

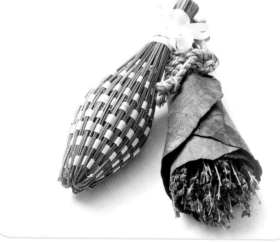

PLANT TIPS

✳ Harvest the flowering heads from mid- to high summer, once the lower petals start to look dry. Choose a warm, sunny day and pick in the morning, after the dew has dried.

✳ Hang lavender stems until dry, then shred the flowerlets into an airtight container and store in a cool, dark place.

USING THE FLOWERS

For insect bites, rub the fresh flowers on to and around a bite; the flowers also deter biting insects.

USING THE ESSENTIAL OIL

If you feel anxious or frazzled, place 2 drops of essential oil of lavender in a vaporiser or a bowl of hot water – studies have shown that exposure to the scent reduces anxiety and lifts mood, as well as producing a significantly improved ability to concentrate. Or, if you become distressed waiting for your doctor or midwife, place 1 drop of the essential oil on a handkerchief and inhale. When you reach the delivery room, use 2 drops of the essential oil in a vaporiser to help to calm your birth attendants as well as you.

For sleeplessness, place a couple of drops of essential oil of lavender in a vaporiser or a bowl of hot water for 30 minutes before bed. Or, take a lavender-scented bath (see opposite) beforehand.

To treat varicose veins, swish 3 drops of essential oil of lavender into a bowl of water then float a flannel on the surface to pick up the oil. Wring out the flannel to make a compress. Elevate your legs and place the compress on them. When the compress has warmed, soak again and repeat.

When your feet are swollen, rest them in a cool footbath containing 2 drops of essential oil of lavender.

LOOKING AHEAD To relieve perineal discomfort in the postnatal period, mix 6 drops of essential oil of lavender in 1 tbsp grapeseed oil and add to your bath.

OFF-THE-SHELF REMEDIES

✳ *Lavandula angustifolia* (also known as English lavender or true lavender) yields the best-quality oil. Search for this name when buying essential oil – it is quite expensive. This is also the species to plant if you want to grow your own.

✳ Avoid oils simply marked as 'lavender oil', that is, with no given botanical name. They are likely to be mixes of the less useful medicinal oils *Lavandula latifolia* (spike or Spanish lavender) and *Lavandula* x *intermedia* (lavandin), the variety used for laundry products.

✳ Look for pillows filled with dried lavender – or make your own – to ease insomnia.

✳ Spritz hot or sun-irritated skin with a lavender hydrosol. This also makes a good hair treatment after rinsing or before heat styling, to add shine.

✳ Lavender is a traditional scent for bed-linen – use lavender water (see page 76) or hydrosol in your iron iron or spritz directly on to linen before ironing. Alternatively, add a few drops of the essential oil or lavender water to the final rinse in the washing machine.

Perineal massage oil

Massaging your perineum – the area of tissue between your vagina and anus – daily from 34 or 35 weeks increases its elasticity and improves blood flow. This makes the tissue more likely to stretch easily (and less painfully) during birth, reducing the likelihood of tears and stitching. A 2006 study found that women who had massaged the perineum were less likely to report pain three months after the birth.

1 tbsp olive oil
1 drop essential oil of lavender

Mix the oils together well. After a bath or shower, when you feel warm and relaxed and the area is soft, sit on a towel and coat your fingers in a little of the oil. Gently insert one or both thumbs just inside your vagina – by about 3 cm – on the back wall. Rest your fingers on your buttocks. Now press down towards your anus and massage by moving your thumbs and forefingers up and out, making a U shape. Repeat for 5 minutes, increasing pressure towards your anus as the action starts to feel more comfortable. Try to relax as you massage.

Lavender bags

Hanging lavender bags from store-bought coat hangers is an easy way to scent the wardrobe in a nursery.

10 cm x 20 cm piece of fine lawn or silky ribbon
20 g dried lavender flowers
20 cm narrow ribbon

Fold the fabric or ribbon in half, right sides together. Leaving 1 cm seam sew up two sides. Turn inside out, pressing out the corner with the point of a scissors or a seam ripper, then iron flat. Fill with lavender flowers, leaving a gap of about 2 cm at the top, then sew the top closed. Tie to the to the coat hanger using a length of narrow ribbon.

Lavender bath

In the early stages of labour a lavender bath can help you to relax and focus. After childbirth, increase the weight of flowers to 100 g. If you don't have time to make the infusion, just add 3–4 drops of essential oil of lavender to the water, and swish well to disperse before stepping in.

20 g dried lavender flowers
2 litres just-boiled water
1 drop essential oil of tea tree (after the birth only)

Place the flowers in a large saucepan and pour over the water. Put on a lid and allow the flowers to steep for at least 20 minutes (overnight gives greatest potency). Strain into the bath.

After the birth, add 250 ml of this infusion to 1 litre of warm water and add the tea tree oil. Use as a soothing wash after you use the toilet.

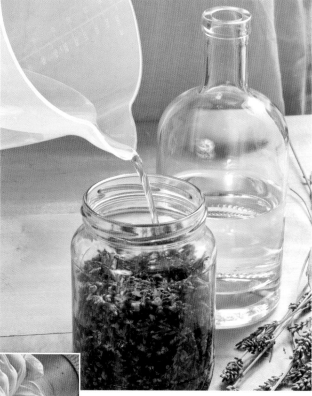

Lavender water

During your third trimester add a little of this uplifting but calming scented water to the final rinse in your washing machine for its clean aroma, use in the iron when pressing bed-linen to encourage sleep, or use to spritz kitchen worktops to kill germs. If you are not using your own lavender grown without pesticides, choose dried organic lavender flowers. You will need a large lidded glass kilner-type jar and a dark glass bottle with a lid.

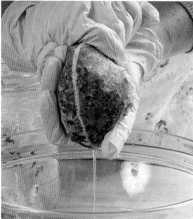

100 g fresh or 50 g dried lavender flowers
250 ml vodka
250 ml distilled water

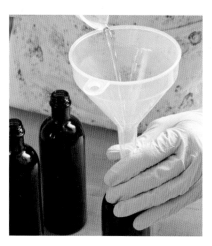

Place the lavender flowers into the large glass jar. Pour over the vodka and then the distilled water, making sure that the flowers are covered by at least 5 cm of liquid. (You may need to add more vodka and water to achieve this.) Lid and leave in a cool, dark place for a month. Shake every few days.

After a month, strain either through a jelly bag (see page 7) squeezing out as much water as possible with your hands, or through a muslin-lined sieve, squeezing as much liquid as possible with the back of a wooden spoon. Discard the muslin and lavender flowers.

Using a funnel, decant the lavender water into the clean, dark glass bottle and lid tightly. Store in a cool, dark place for up to a year.

To use, pour into the reservoir of your iron, add to the washing machine before the final rinse, or decant into a spritzer bottle and top up with water. Shake before spraying.

Alfalfa

strengthening, boosting immunity

The name of this plant derives from the Arabic *al-fasfasah*, meaning 'father of all foods' because it contains more protein than any other crop used to feed livestock.

When eaten as a food, the young leaves and shoots of this perennial plant (*Medicago sativa*) help to build an overall feeling of good health if you're feeling fatigued or under the weather. This traditional fodder plant, used fresh or dried, stimulates the appetite and supplies many of the nutrients needed to beat common deficiencies – it has been used for years to support convalescence, treat anaemia and as a tonic for the immune system.

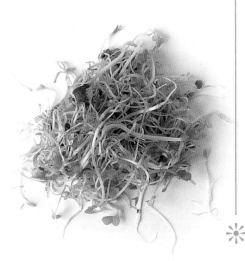

Alfalfa is a mild diuretic and liver cleanser, and is used in Ayurvedic medicine to treat fluid retention. Nutritionally, the leaves and shoots of the alfalfa plant are rich in easily absorbed vitamins – beta-carotene, B vitamins including folate, and vitamins C and K. The latter is particularly useful in pregnancy because it supports blood-clotting, and so may help to reduce postnatal bleeding. The plant is also rich in protein – the leaves contain eight essential amino acids – and many more minerals than other grains. It is particularly high in calcium, phosphorus, iron, and fluorides,

useful to protect the teeth. Its phytonutrients include chlorophyll and antioxidant tricin. This makes a little alfalfa especially valuable in the last few weeks if your diet isn't as good as it could be.

PLANT TIPS

* This is an edible wild plant; you can find it growing on roadsides and at the edges of arable fields, where it has naturalised after being sown as a fodder plant. Take an identification guide when picking from the wild.

* You can look for alfalfa plants to raise at home at farmer's markets and plant sales. Make sure they look bright and crisp; don't buy plants that are starting to turn brown or running to seed.

CAUTION Raw seeds are an abortifacient – always sprout before eating. Raw or lightly cooked sprouted seeds carry a risk of salmonella contamination. Avoid alfalfa if you have an auto-immune condition, such as multiple sclerosis, lupus or rheumatoid arthritis. Avoid if you take blood-thinning medication such as warfarin.

USING THE HERB

In food eat the young leaves in salads for their good amounts of vitamin K.

To add interest to a room the lilac-blue flowers (similar to a wild sweet pea or lupin (the plant belongs to the pea family).have a country chic appeal when bunched in a jug.

For a jaded appetite and/or constipation a cup of alfalfa tea (from the dried leaves) is said to be particularly stimulating and has a slight laxative effect. Don't drink more than 1 cup daily.

To soothe dry or sun-damaged skin, try alfalfa honey moisturiser (see opposite).

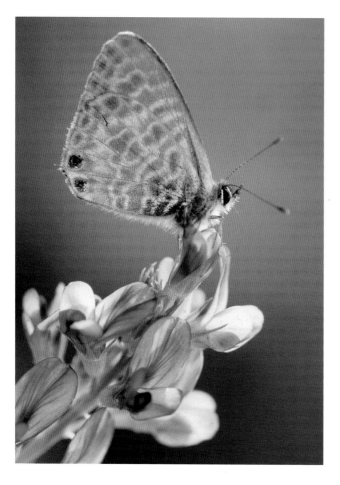

NATURAL GARDEN FERTILISER

If you have a neglected plot which needs a fertility boost, sow perennial alfalfa seed in spring or autumn as a green manure, or soil conditioner, and leave in situ for two years to fix nitrogen into the soil and increase the yield of successive crops. After year one the plant will flourish, giving masses more alfalfa than you can eat. This crop likes a light soil and will tolerate cold and drought.

LOOKING AHEAD To rebuild your energy levels after the birth, add raw or lightly cooked sprouted seeds to salads and sandwiches, burgers and falafel. Soak the dried seeds overnight, then drain and place somewhere dark, rinsing daily until they begin to sprout (5–6 days). They are safe to eat once the sprout has set two leaves.

To encourage lactation, eat sprouted seeds as above or buy alfalfa seed tea. Be aware that the oestrogen-like effects of the constituent isoflavones and coumarins mean that when taken in large amounts alfalfa can decrease the effectiveness of birth-control pills.

OFF-THE-SHELF REMEDIES

✳ Alfalfa juice is said to be good for maintaining thick glossy hair and preventing hair loss after the birth. On its own, alfalfa juice is quite bitter, so search out vegetable juices containing alfalfa in the mix – it's often blended with carrot and lettuce. Blend together alfalfa juice and fresh cucumber to dab on to skin breakouts for its astringent effect.

✳ Alfalfa powder is available at health stores or online as a food supplement. Add 1 tsp of the powder to clay masks for its high vitamin and mineral content.

✳ Look for alfalfa extract (*Medicago sativa* on the ingredients list) in beauty products; this is used for its antioxidant properties, to boost collagen production and aid firmness, and in products for very dry skin, such as Clarins' HydraQuench Intensive Serum and Extra-Firming Night Cream.

❋ Alfalfa honey – from the flowers – has a lightly spiced mild flavour and can be less sweet than some honeys.

❋ Add alfalfa meal to soaps for its exfoliating power.

Alfalfa-honey moisturising treatment

Alfalfa extract is used in beauty products to soothe dryness, heal sun damage and condition the skin. This oil feels good if your skin is tight or itchy. All types of honey are humectant, helping to retain moisture and elasticity.

2 tbsp alfalfa honey
2 tbsp grapeseed oil
1 tsp lemon juice

Mix together all the ingredients until they are well combined. Massage over areas of dry skin, especially your elbows, knees, sun-damaged shoulders and around stretchmarks. Ask someone to do your feet, focusing on your heels. Then rinse off by stepping into a bath (add another 25 g honey, if you prefer, as you add the hot water) or rinse off with a hot flannel.

Alfalfa soap balls

The saponins found in plants are added to shampoos and cleansers for their natural foaming action. (Only alfalfa leaf foams, so be sure to buy leaf powder.) Soapmakers use alfalfa powder for its natural green colour and gentle abrasive quality. This soap is made with easy-to-use soap flakes; choose castille soap flakes milled using olive oil or grate a bar of castille soap.

MAKES 12 SMALL OR 8 LARGE BALLS

350 g castille soap flakes
5 tbsp orange flower water or hydrosol
5 tbsp olive oil, plus extra for coating
2 drops essential oil of tangerine
1 tbsp honey
1 tsp alfalfa leaf powder
4 tbsp dried rose petals, crushed

Put the soap flakes in a large mixing bowl, add the flower water or hydrosol, and stir. Add the oils, stir again, then mix in the honey and leaf powder.

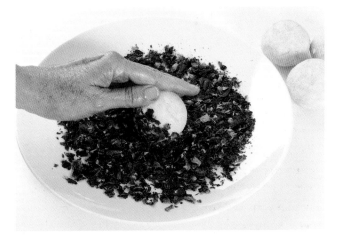

Knead the mixture until you have a smooth dough, then separate into 8–12 sections. Scoop out each section with a spoon and roll between your oiled palms until smooth.

Scatter the rose petals over a large plate, moisten the palms of your hands with olive oil, roll the balls between your palms to coat them with a little oil, then roll in the petals. Place on baking parchment and allow to dry in a cool place for about a week. The balls will start to lose their scent and petal colour after about three months.

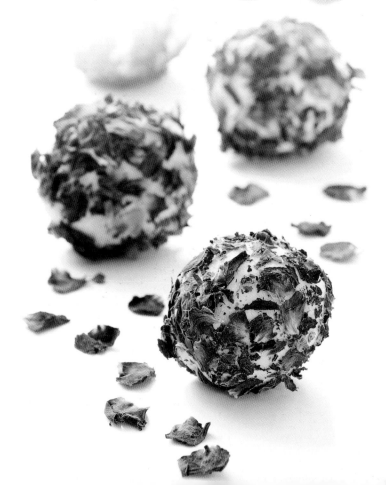

Orange flower

lifting anxiety, restoring calm

Orange blossom forms part of fertility celebrations in many traditions, not least in bridal crowns and bouquets, reputedly to calm the nerves. It is connected with the Greek goddess of earth and fertility Gaia, or mother earth.

The delicately perfumed white blossom of the bitter orange tree (*Citrus aurantium*) is associated with fullness and fertility – perhaps because the tree bears fruit, flowers and foliage all at the same time. The leaves, flowers and peel contain a volatile oil which has anti-inflammatory, antibacterial and antifungal properties, while the fruit is used across the globe to stimulate digestion, relieve flatulence and ease constipation.

Nutritionally, oranges are valued for their folate and immune-boosting vitamin C and have long been used to ease coughs and colds – and to make tangy marmalade. Neroli oil is a very expensive essential oil distilled from the flowers of the bitter orange. The more woody, floral-scented (and cheaper) petitgrain oil is distilled from the leaves, young shoots and unripe fruit. The leaves and flowers have sedative properties, and their oils and flower waters have a calming and rebalancing effect on the nervous system. Neroli, in particular, is uplifting and promotes sleep. In 2000, a study found that diffusing orange oil in a dentist's waiting room decreased levels of anxiety in women patients; neroli and petitgrain can also lower the heart rate and prevent palpitations. These orange

CAUTION Petitgrain oil is phototoxic; do not expose your skin to sunlight after use. (The constituent bergapten is often added to self-tanning preparations to encourage skin pigmentation.) Neroli oil is not phototoxic.

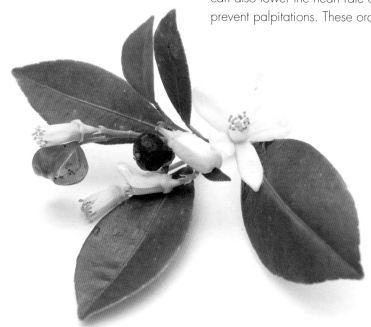

oils are especially useful for skin problems, boosting circulation and having antifungal and antibacterial properties. Neroli oil is valued by aromatherapists for its regenerative effect on the skin, which helps to combat stretchmarks; petitgrain is recommended for oily skin.

USING THE HERB

As a toner after cleansing or if you feel hot, use refrigerated orange-blossom water or hydrosol.

When life feels overwhelming, add 4 drops of essential oil of neroli to the water in a vaporiser. For a more subtle aroma, substitute a little orange-blossom water or hydrosol. This can have a valuable tranquilising effect during labour, too. Making a pomander (see over) may help lift your spirits late on in pregnancy.

As a relaxant and restorative, try a whole-body or foot massage using oranges or orange-scented products (see page 82).

For a restorative skin treatment, add 1 drop of either neroli or petitgrain oil to a facial sauna. To treat stretchmarks, massage in the blend on page 82.

For a relaxing and skin-softening bath, add 4 drops of essential oil of neroli to 1 tbsp full-fat milk and swish into a bath. If you have the energy, add the zest of 2 Seville oranges (place a strainer over the plug hole when you let the water out, to catch the zest).

To ease insomnia, place 1 drop of neroli oil on your pillow, or spritz the air around your bed with a hydrosol. Alternatively, you can steep 1 tsp of dried orange-flower blossom in just-boiled water and sip before bed to soothe the digestive tract and bring on sleep.

To combat energy dips, eat a whole orange – the pectin (a form of soluble fibre) is effective in stabilising blood-sugar levels. Or fragrance your room with essential oil of sweet orange (*Citrus sinensis*); its cheerful brightness is useful for boosting energy in these last long weeks. If you have a potted orange tree, stroke the leaves to release the scent.

For pregnancy constipation, drink freshly squeezed juice, bits and all, topped up with a little water. A daily glass of orange juice is all you need to meet your extra vitamin C requirements in pregnancy.

During labour, to help prevent shallow breathing during transition, add 2 drops of neroli oil to a vaporiser. Alternatively, substitute 1 drop each of frankincense and rose, for their calming effect.

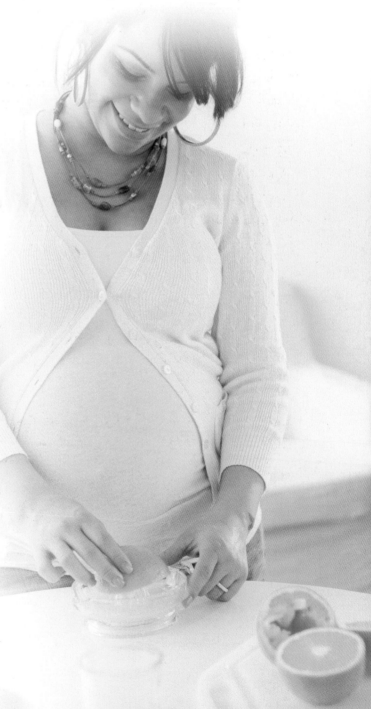

MAKING POMANDERS

The scent of orange and clove oils is uplifting when you feel heavy and lethargic towards the end of your pregnancy. Clove oil is said to be pain-relieving during childbirth, but is not recommended during pregnancy, so instead use the spice to make pomanders, a traditional way to employ the insect-repellent and bactericidal properties of cloves. Simply take 2 or 3 heavy oranges (the heavier the fruit, the more juice) and a bag of whole cloves. Stud each orange all over with cloves (choose the ones with buds still attached to the spikes), puncturing the flesh with the pointed end and making a pattern as you work. Either place in a bowl to scent the room or tie with ribbon and hang up.

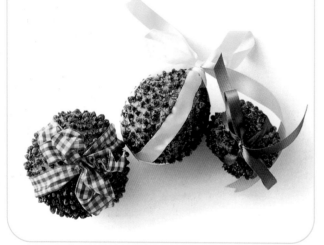

OFF-THE-SHELF REMEDIES
* Buy fresh bitter oranges and preserve their goodness for use later in the year by making masses of tangy marmalade. Don't try to eat the flesh raw; these oranges are beyond tart! Look for Seville oranges – available for a few short weeks in late winter.
* Look out for candied peel of bitter or Seville orange, for use in cakes and tarts.
* It's important to use fresh essential oils of citrus fruit (check the best-by date) and to store them in dark glass bottles in a cool place, to preserve their active ingredients.

* Neroli oil is one of the most expensive essential oils, since the yield is so low. Check for the botanical name *Citrus aurantium* to be sure yours is a pure oil. The best oils come from France.
* Petitgrain is a traditional ingredient of eau de Cologne – keep a blend in your bag and use a quick splash as a pick-me-up. The best petitgrain oil comes from France and southern Italy.
* Neroli hydrosol is more medicinally useful than a flower water. Because it is a 'distillate' – the aromatic water left over after the essential oil has been extracted from a plant by water or steam distillation – it contains all the water-soluble active ingredients of the plant. Some say the scent is more redolent of orange blossom than essential oil of neroli.
* Check the ingredients list of orange-blossom waters – some are made using synthetic flavourings and alcohol; these have no therapeutic value. Orange blossom is also a component of Hungary Water, made by macerating herbs including rosemary, sage and lemon balm with cider vinegar. Use on cottonwool to deal with pimples or as a toner to refresh areas of greasy skin.
* Use culinary-grade orange-blossom water to scent cakes, biscuits, custards and couscous.
* Orange-blossom honey is good both for eating and in skincare preparations.

Relaxing orange-flower massage oil
Essential oil of neroli calms the nervous system, soothes digestive ailments and promotes deep sleep. The frankincense oil deepens the breathing to bring about a sense of great calm. Use this blend in the bath in the final weeks if worries about the birth stop you from sleeping.

1 tbsp grapeseed oil
2 drops essential oil of neroli
1 drop essential oil of frankincense

Mix all the oils together and swish into a warm bath just before stepping in. Relax in the bath focusing your thoughts on the calm and regular movement of your breath, cool as it comes in through your nostrils and warm as you exhale. It can help to count your breath in for 3 or

4 and out for the same length of time. Lengthen the count as you feel yourself relaxing. This calming technique can be useful during the early stages of labour, too.

Rosehip and orange stretchmark blend

Neroli and petitgrain oils are skin-soothing, while the other oils in this blend are useful for healing damaged skin. Bach Flowers olive remedy helps with extreme physical tiredness. Don't expose your bump to the sun after using this blend if you make it with petitgrain oil, which can make the skin photosensitive.

1 tbsp olive oil
1 tsp rosehip oil
1 tsp wheatgerm oil
2 drops Bach Flower Remedy Olive®
4 drops essential oil of neroli or petitgrain

Mix the oils together, then whisk in the Bach Flower drops until well combined. Drop in the essential oils, mix well and rub into your belly, thighs and breasts. Alternatively, swish into the bath just before stepping in.

Orange foot massage treatment

The cheerful scent of this foot rub is just the thing when you can no longer see your feet. Needless to say, someone has to give this treatment to you, which is why it is so relaxing and uplifting! You will need a footbath (or bucket) and a couple of old towels (the whole thing can get a bit messy).

2 large oranges
1 tbsp honey
1 tbsp grapeseed oil
4 drops essential oil of neroli or petitgrain

Juice and zest the oranges into a bowl, picking out and discarding any pips. Stir in the honey. In another, smaller bowl, stir together the grapeseed and essential oils.

Soak your feet in a warm footbath for 5 minutes, then have your partner dry your feet and massage the orange-honey mixture into your feet, especially around areas of hard skin. Place your feet up on a towel and rest for another 5 minutes to allow the oranges and honey to carry out their softening and moisturising work. Plunge your feet into the footbath to rinse off, and dry again.

Ask your partner to massage the scented oil into each foot in turn for another 5 minutes, working around each of the toes, up the sole and sweeping around your ankles, until your feet feel rested and smooth, and are sweetly scented.

Five-flower remedy

stress-busting, calming

Star of Bethlehem, a member of the lily family, has a white line down the midrib of each leaf, resembling a reverse linea negra, the dark line that commonly runs down the abdomen of pregnant women.

Busy Lizzie
Flowers of Impatiens walleriana to ease impatience and calm agitation.

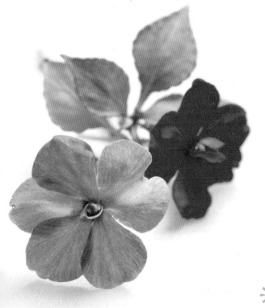

A blend of five Bach Flower Remedies, Rescue Remedy© is just the thing to rely on in an emergency or time of stress, so it is perfect to keep in your birth bag in anticipation of the big day. And if the very thought of the birth makes you feel fearful or panicky, the remedy is useful well in advance, too. Bach Flower Remedies were developed by the Harley Street consultant and bacteriologist Dr Edward Bach in the 1920s and 30s, and he recommended particular remedies to treat different mental or emotional imbalances, so enhancing general well-being.

Bach Flower Remedies are made by floating flowerheads in sunlit water, or by boiling woodier plants then mixing the brew with alcohol to make a mother tincture, which is further diluted for sale. Five-flower or Rescue Remedy© is made up of five separate remedies that together encourage inner calm, focus and control. The five flowers are Rock Rose for calmness and courage, Cherry Plum for self-control, Clematis for faintness, Star of Bethlehem for shock and to help you cope with the unexpected, and *Impatiens* (busy lizzie) for agitation and impatience. As the big day draws near, all of these attributes will help to keep you on an even keel.

Since the remedies are made using brandy, always dilute in water for use in pregnancy.

USING THE REMEDY

In cooking busy Lizzie flowers (*Impatiens wallerana*) are edible and have a sweet flavour. Use them as a garnish in salads or freeze in ice-cube trays to float in drinks.

To calm jangly nerves, try making up a batch of the lip balm on page 86 and using whenever necessary.

To create a positive atmosphere in the birthing room, making it more conducive to labouring, make up a spray using the five essential oils (see page 86).

OFF-THE-SHELF REMEDIES

For reassurance about the provenance of remedies, look for the Dr Bach signature on the glass bottle. This guarantees that a remedy derives from a mother tincture prepared by the Bach Centre in Mount Vernon in Oxfordshire, UK.

❋ Place 4 drops of Rescue Remedy© in a glass of water and sip as required. Keep the glass in the refrigerator until you feel you need another sip. Make up a fresh glass each morning. In extreme situations, make sure your partner knows to put 4 drops on to your tongue directly from the bottle. Your partner might find that this remedy calms his nerves, too!

❋ Add 4 drops of the remedy to a cold compress and ask your birth partner to use to mop your brow during labour.

❋ A Rescue Remedy© spray may be most convenient during the birth – before the big day show your partner how to administer 2 sprays on to your tongue.

❋ Rescue Remedy© pastilles are free from sugar and alcohol and good to suck during long labours – choose from elderflower and orange or blackcurrant flavours.

❋ If congestion makes it increasingly hard to breathe through your nose, lips can get chapped in the weeks leading up to the birth and during labour. Look for a lip balm made using Rescue Remedy© or make the lip balm on page 86.

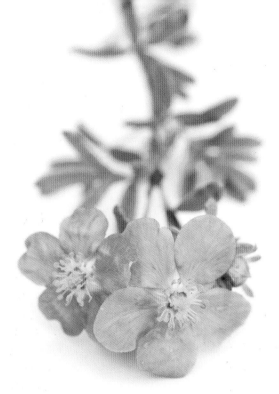

Rock rose
Flowers of the Cistaceae family induce feelings of calm and courage.

❋ Rescue Remedy© cream, made with crab apple in the mix, can be rubbed into your temples and hands – ask your partner to do this during labour. This is also good for bruising after the birth. Ask your partner to massage the cream into your shoulders next day if you spent hours in labour pushing against a wall, the back of the bed or the side of the bath.

You can take the remedies in the Rescue formula individually, too. The following are particularly useful in the weeks leading up to the birth.

❋ Impatiens if you feel irritated by waiting in the last trimester and just want to get on with it, or feel agitated or held back by others' more methodical behaviour at this time.

❋ Rock Rose for the kind of panicky fear that makes it difficult to think straight.

❋ Cherry Plum if you worry about losing control or acting out of character during the birth.

❋ Clematis to anchor you in the present if daydreaming about the future is preventing you from attending to day-to-day realities or you feel fuzzy-brained.

❋ Try Walnut, too, during labour; this remedy aids transition of all forms, encouraging constant forward movement of both contractions and baby.

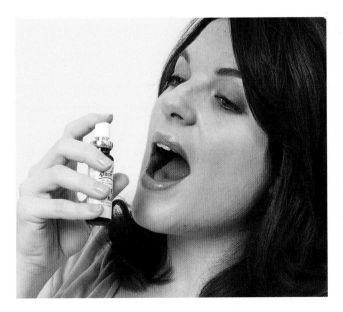

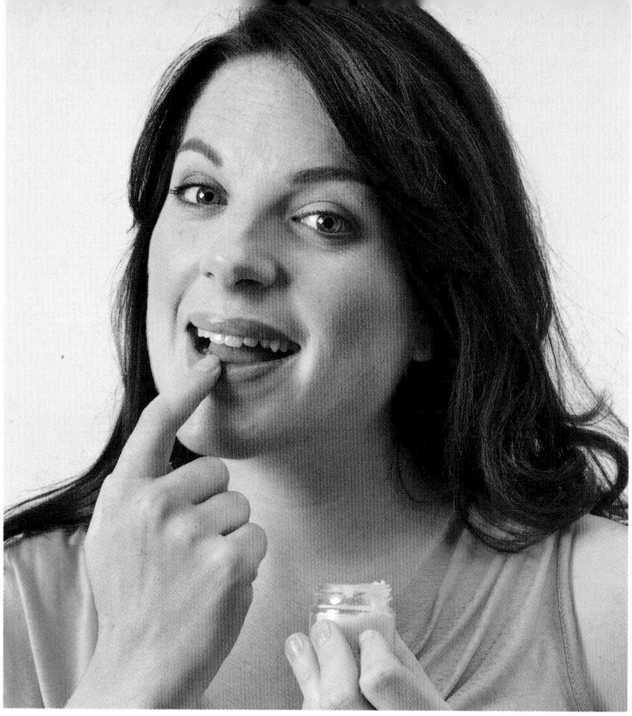

- If the birth leaves you feeling traumatised physically or emotionally, and you seek consolation, take Star of Bethlehem.
- Individual remedies diluted in a glycerine-water mix in 10 ml dropper bottles are available if you prefer alcohol-free remedies; contact The Bach Centre online (www.bachcentre.com).

Floral lip balm

This creamy balm only takes 10 minutes to make and its vanilla scent is a welcome floral pick-me-up at this stressful time. You will need one 30 ml or two 15 ml sterilised glass jars with lids.

1 tsp beeswax, grated
1 tsp cocoa butter
½ tsp honey
4 tsp sweet almond or argan oil
2 drops Rescue Remedy©
1 vitamin E capsule
¼ tsp vanilla extract

Place a heatproof bowl over a pan of simmering water. Place the beeswax, cocoa butter and honey in the bowl and heat until completely melted. Remove the bowl from the heat. Add the oil and Rescue Remedy©, stirring well until emulsified, then squeeze in the capsule and stir again. Finally stir in the vanilla extract. Spoon into the jar(s) and leave to cool and set before putting on the lid(s). This will keep, refrigerated, for about three months.

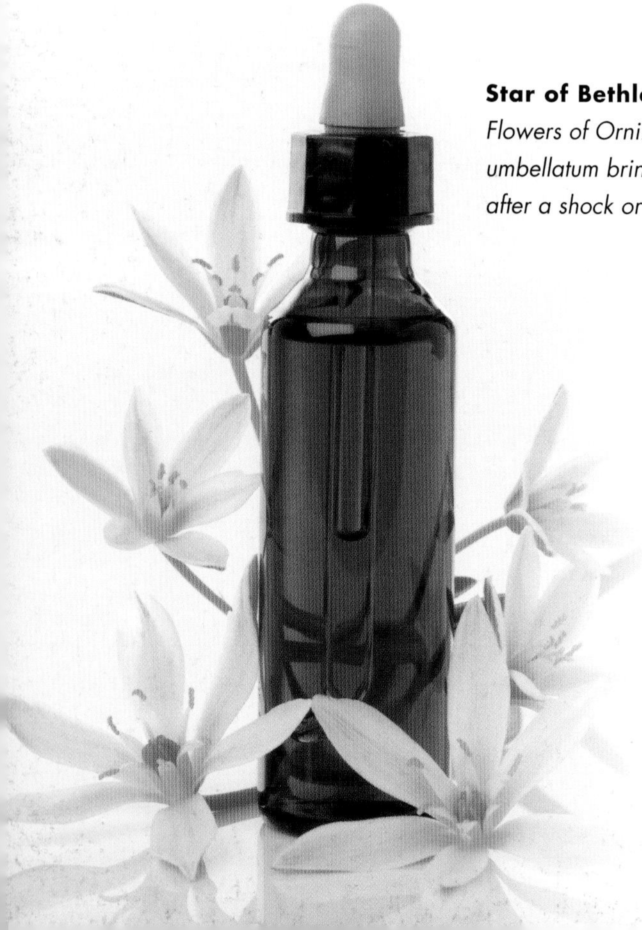

Star of Bethlehem
Flowers of Ornithogalum umbellatum bring comfort after a shock or trauma.

Birth room spray

This five-flower scented spray can be used to freshen the room and bed-linen – it cancels out the institutional smell of hospitals. Rose has a relaxing, opening effect, lavender is calming, geranium uplifting, jasmine strengthens contractions and neroli is steadying for the nerves. If you find five aromas overwhelming, just use your favourite two or three; experiment a few days in advance. You will need a 100 ml bottle with a pump-action spray top.

2 tsp vodka
3 drops essential oil of geranium
1 drop essential oil of jasmine
1 drop essential oil of rose
2 drops essential oil of lavender
1 drop essential oil of neroli
80 ml distilled water

Place the vodka in the bottle and drop in your preferred combination of essential oils. Stir to combine. Add the water, put on the top and shake vigorously before use.

Part 6
HEALING POSTNATAL HERBS

Herbs to help you adjust to change, for recuperation
and to generate a plentiful supply of milk

Arnica

countering shock, relieving pain and swelling

Homeopaths say that women who stoically say 'I'm fine' after birth need the remedy Arnica more than those who display more overt symptoms of shock.

When dried, the golden yellow, daisy-like flowers, roots and rhizomes of the perennial mountain plant *Arnica montana* are considered a useful first-aid herb in the aftermath of a shock to the body which also affects the emotions. The mountain daisy is perhaps best known in its homeopathic form, as the remedy to turn to after trauma, injury or surgery – it's often referred to as the homeopathic painkiller.

A 2005 trial in Jerusalem found that taking the homeopathic remedies Arnica and Bellis perennis together after giving birth – as compared with a placebo – seemed to reduce postnatal blood loss. Arnica is also recommended by herbalists in ointment and compress form, as an external treatment for the bruising and muscular aches that can result from over-exertion. Many new mothers would include childbirth in that description!

The herb is thought to speed healing by increasing local blood supply, reducing inflammation and bruising, dispersing trapped fluids and arresting bleeding, also easing the pain that can accompany such symptoms. That said, in a clinical trial in 2010, using arnica cream on calves that ached after exercise actually increased leg pain 24 hours later. Arnica is also valued by herbalists for bringing the nervous system back into balance.

The plant is often recommended as a hair conditioner, and is reputed to increase hair growth – useful if there now seem to be an alarming number of hairs in your brush in the morning. The plant variety used in hair preparations may be the close relation of the mountain daisy, *A. angustifolia alpina*.

CAUTION If you are allergic to ragweed and plants in the daisy family Compositae (Asteraceae), you may react to this herb, too. Do not apply to broken skin. Do not apply compresses or creams to nipples while breastfeeding.

PLANT TIPS

✳ This is not a plant you should try to harvest yourself because of the risk of contact dermatitis; it's safest to buy ready-prepared tincture, homeopathic remedies and flower essences.

USING THE HERB

For recovery from shock and battered post-birth feelings, especially after a first baby, take the homeopathic remedy Arnica in the 200c potency as soon as possible after delivery – be sure to pack some in your birth bag. Dissolve 1 pill under your tongue three times a day, until symptoms subside. Give some to your exhausted partner, too. (For a deep-healing homeopathic combination see page 90.)

If your bed feels too hard, homeopathic Arnica is the remedy for you – homeopaths use this symptom as a guide to prescribing an appropriate remedy.

To combat feelings of unreality, common after the experience of labour, Arnica flower essence is believed to help reintegrate body and emotions.

For stiff or aching muscles, in the legs and shoulders, particularly after a long labour spent squatting or leaning forwards, apply arnica ointment two or three times daily. It is especially effective for bruising and swelling. Alternatively, apply the compress on page 90.

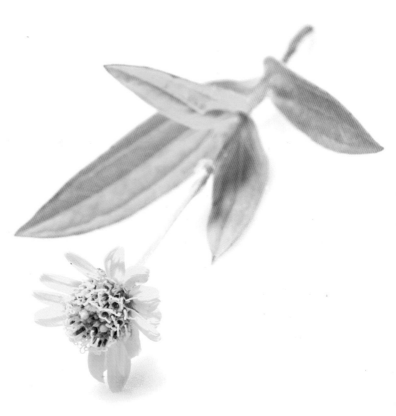

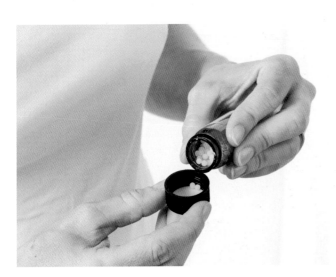

For aching feet, place 10 drops of arnica tincture into a warm footbath and swish well to disperse before soaking your feet.

OFF-THE-SHELF REMEDIES

✳ Arnica is available as a flower essence made from North American varieties of the herb. Look for the botanical names *A. mollis* and *A. chamissonis*. It is also available in blends. The blend containing yarrow (*Achillea millefolium*) is thought to fortify those who feel wounded and vulnerable (yarrow is known as the warrior's herb). Place 4 drops of a flower essence in a glass of water and sip through the day, or in emergencies drop directly on to your tongue. Your partner might benefit, too.

✳ When taking homeopathic Arnica – and homeopathic remedies in general – it's best not to eat or drink anything for 15–20 minutes before or afterwards. Avoid brushing your teeth, too (mint may neutralise the remedy) and try not to touch the remedy with your hands. Tip one pill into the cap of the remedy phial and drop it beneath your tongue.

✳ Choose arnica creams and ointments made with soothing natural ingredients such as shea butter rather than petroleum-based ingredients. Nelson's products are reliably good (see page 125) – look for their Arnicare brand.

✳ If you lack the time to make an arnica compress, buy one of Dr Hauschka's ready-packed ones (see page 125).

✳ Arnica has been used in trials for hair loss, If you would like to try this for yourself, check the label of scalp massage products, shampoos and conditioners for the term *A. montana* in the ingredients list.

Arnica combination remedy

To replicate the Jerusalem study on postnatal blood loss (see page 88), take homeopathic Arnica with the homeopathic remedy Bellis perennis after delivery. Bellis perennis is derived from the common daisy and is recommended for healing deep-tissue injuries, especially after a caesarean or forceps delivery.

homeopathic Arnica 30c
homeopathic Bellis perennis 30c

Take 4 Arnica pills and 4 Bellis perennis pills immediately after delivery if you can, dissolving them under your tongue. Then repeat as you need relief, every two hours if necessary, until symptoms improve.

Stop taking the Arnica pills after 48 hours, but continue taking the Bellis perennis three times a day between meals, until you have stopped bleeding.

Arnica compress

Make this compress to apply to sore muscles or bruising, but never use over broken or damaged skin. Do not apply to the skin for longer than six hours per day. You will need a clean flannel.

1 tsp arnica tincture
250 ml tepid water

In a bowl, dilute the tincture in the water, stirring until well combined. Wet the flannel, then squeeze out and apply gently to the affected area. Leave in place for 15 minutes as you relax. Relaxation after childbirth is the best way to promote healing.
in hair

Arnica and hair loss
Regular use of arnica in hair products is reputed to strengthen the hair, preventing or reducing post-pregnancy hair loss and keeping hair healthy. Use a wide-toothed comb to avoid snagging fragile hair.

Pot marigold

healing wounds, soothing pain

Some say this flower is associated with motherhood because its name recalls the perfection of the Virgin Mary.

The vivid yellow-orange petals and flowerheads of pot marigold *(Calendula officinalis)* are valued for soothing irritated, inflamed skin and healing cuts, grazes, wounds and bruising. This herb has an astringent action, and its antiseptic and antimicrobial properties help to guard against infection after childbirth. It also has an anti-inflammatory action, eases muscle spasms and may stimulate the immune system. Marigold is considered a women's reproductive herb, as it is used to treat pain and cramps or regulate and stem bleeding. But after childbirth, calendula is perhaps most valued for healing sore or cracked nipples.

USING THE HERB

To ward off the baby blues, use the flowers in a relaxing bath (see page 93) or plant up in pots and pop on a windowsill – looking at the yellow-orange rays of the marigold is said to be a tonic for the eyes. The herbalists Culpeper and Gerard valued the plant for comforting the heart and raising the spirits.

In cooking, add the young leaves and the petals to salads for their bright colour and pungent spiciness or use the petals as a substitute for saffron in rice dishes.

CAUTION If you are allergic to ragweed and plants in the daisy family, you may also be allergic to calendula. Do not combine this plant with sedative medication.

To ease perineal pain or soreness, use the dried flowers in a sitz bath or a tincture as a spray (see page 93).

For indigestion and heartburn, sip a cup of calendula tea.

OFF-THE-SHELF REMEDIES

✳ The homeopathic remedy Calendula is considered an antiseptic and is recommended for healing episiotomies, tears and stitches in the perineum. Use 6x potency.

✳ A little calendula infusion added to a flannel soaked in hot water then squeezed out can be applied to the perineum as a soothing compress.

✳ Use calendula cream for relieving the pain of cracked or sore nipples: 1994 research confirmed its efficacy. Look for calendula nipple creams free from scents (including essential oils), lanolin, petrochemicals and parabens (butyl, propyl and ethyl are names to avoid). Granary Herbs cream is effective, using organic herbs in a simple base; Earth Mama Angel Baby Natural Nipple Butter combines the herb with emollient cocoa butter, shea butter and mango butter.

✳ Weleda's calendula bath for (older) babies is calming for you too before bed. Follow with a massage with calendula oil.

✳ Calendula tincture used neat can be dabbed on with cottonwool to help clear spots. Calendula tincture diluted with two parts water can be used as a mouthwash when you don't have time to brush your teeth and if your gums are sore or bleeding.

✳ Calendula ointment or nappy-rash cream applied at nappy changes will promote healing.

Marigold and lemon balm bath

Petals of marigold and lemon balm are here combined for their ability to 'make the mind and heart merry' as Culpeper noted, as well as for their heady scent. This floral bath is a great way to unwind once your baby is settled for the night. If you don't want to gather up the petals after your bath, tie them in a square of muslin or use a strainer to prevent them from blocking the drain.

25 g dried marigold flowers (*Calendula officinalis*)
25 g dried lemon balm (*Melissa officinalis*)
1tsp grapeseed oil

GROW YOUR OWN

First check the seed or plant name – to benefit from the medicinal properties you need to grow *Calendula officinalis* not more showy plants from the Tagetes species (African or French marigolds). Pot marigolds are easy to raise. Cultivate them from seed in the autumn, indoors in a tray filled with a standard seed compost. Place the seeds about 2 cm apart in the tray, water gently, then wait for them to germinate (they prefer a temperature of around 19°C/66°F). When the seedlings have about six 'true' leaves (the initial two leaves don't count), transfer to individual pots filled with potting compost. In the spring, place the pots outside during the day to acclimatise or 'harden off', then once all danger of frost is over, plant in a sunny position outdoors (or in a windowbox) at least 30 cm apart. Harvest the flowerheads in summer in the morning, once the petals have opened and the dew has dried. Deadhead plants throughout the summer to prolong flowering.

Place the herbs in the bath and fill the bath about halfway with scalding hot water. Leave for 10 minutes to infuse then add cool water until it's a comfortable temperature. Just before stepping in, pour in the oil and swish with your fingers to disperse.

Recline in the bath for 20 minutes, if you can, inhaling the uplifting scent. Now go to bed, if baby allows.

Marigold and sea salt sitz bath

This feels soothing, and encourages the healing of tears, cuts and general soreness and swelling around the perineum. You will need a small plastic basin or portable sitz bath. If you feel strong, try a cold water bath, said to relieve pain more effectively.

100 g dried marigold flowers (*Calendula officinalis*)
4 tbsp sea salt
1 litre boiling water
3 drops essential oil of lavender

Place the dried flowers and sea salt in a large jug and pour over the water. Allow to steep for an hour then strain into the basin and top up with warm water. Add the essential oil, stirring well to disperse. Sit in the water for 10–15 minutes, or soak a clean flannel in the water and use as a compress. Repeat daily.

Healing marigold spray

Keep this powerfully antiseptic potion in the fridge for cool relief. You will need a clean dark glass bottle with a pump-action spray.

50 ml bottle marigold tincture (1:4)
120 ml water

Add 10 drops of the tincture to the water and decant into the bottle. Refrigerate, and spray on the perineum for soothing relief. ('Neat' tincture stings but is more potently antiseptic.) Make up a new bottle after three days.

Calendula ointment

This is a soothing lotion for nappy rash. It contains no water, which irritates nappy rash, and it forms a protective layer on the skin surface. You will need an ovenproof bowl with a lid and two 250 ml sterilised glass jars with lids.

25 g beeswax, grated
250 ml extra-virgin olive oil
50 g dried or 125 g fresh calendula flowers

Place the grated beeswax in an ovenproof bowl. Suspend over a pan of simmering water, add the olive oil and stir until all the wax has dissolved into the oil. Remove the bowl from the heat, stir in the flowers, and put on the lid. Place in a low oven (140°C/275°F/gas mark 1) for three hours, then pour through a muslin-lined sieve into a bowl, pressing with the back of a wooden spoon to extract as much oil as possible.

Decant into the jars while warm and, once cool, put on the lids. Label and date, and store in a cool, dark place. To use, smear over rashes and inflamed skin. This will keep for up to three months.

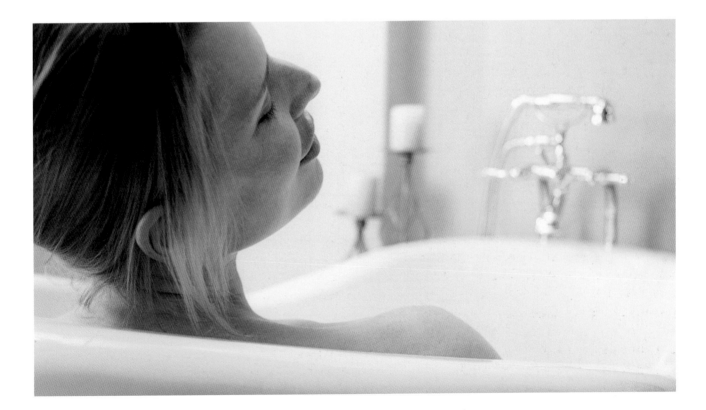

Fennel

calming the stomach, stimulating breast milk

Fennel was once woven into a wreath to crown those who had triumphed after strenuous effort; it was reputed to renew strength, courage and vigour.

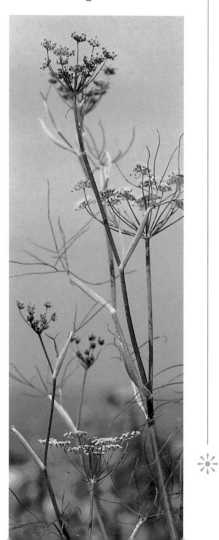

The oval seeds of the fennel plant (*Foeniculum vulgare*) are valued after childbirth for supporting digestion and stimulating milk supply. The volatile oil in the seeds has carminative properties, expelling wind and reducing bloating and its antispasmodic action settles the pain that can accompany these symptoms; it also stimulates the appetite. It doesn't just work on mothers: midwives and herbalists often recommend fennel for its calming effect on young babies with colic. The bulb of Florence fennel (*F. vulgare azoricum*), which shares some of these properties, can be eaten raw or cooked and has a delicious aniseed-like flavour that marries well with fish.

In Ayurvedic medicine wind and cramping are considered common postnatal symptoms, caused by excess vata. This is one of the body's three energies and is concentrated in the abdominal and pelvic region – and after the birth an excess of this energy is thought to be aggravated by interrupted sleep, an ever-changing daily schedule and all that newly acquired space in the abdominal area.

In many herbal traditions, fennel is regarded as cleansing and antiseptic, and is used as a tonic for the kidneys, liver and spleen; it is also associated with the bladder. The diuretic properties of fennel are useful for treating water retention and it can also ease the difficult or burning urination of cystitis. After the birth fennel can ease menstrual-like after-pains.

Above all, however, fennel is famed for boosting the flow of milk in nursing mothers – these qualities have been described since ancient Greek times. By drinking fennel tea breastfeeding mothers easily pass on the colic-calming properties of the seeds to their babies. Fennel has long been considered an aid to weight loss – and herbalist and diarist John Evelyn wrote that it 'recreates the brain', also desirable after pregnancy!

CAUTION Avoid large doses of fennel if you have epilepsy.

USING THE HERB

As a digestif, chew on fennel seeds after a rich meal. Or make the seed mix on page 97 to finish a meal.

To counter rich foods, use fennel oil in dressings and marinades (see recipe on page 96) or stuff gutted fish with the chopped leaves and stalks.

To combat wind and bloating, place ¼–½ tsp of fennel seeds in a mug and pour over boiling water. Leave to infuse for 5–10 minutes, then strain and sip. If you like the flavour of lemon balm, try the tea blend on page 96, or substitute a little fresh ginger root, grated.

To treat colic, drink one cup of fennel seed tea up to six times a day if you are breastfeeding.

To aid milk production and to tempt a jaded appetite, add fennel seeds to cake mixes for snacks .

Exploit the expectorant properties of fennel if you have a phlegmy cough: gargle with an infusion of the seeds. Place 1 tsp in a pan with 750 ml water and simmer for 20–30 minutes, until reduced to about 500 ml. This also works as a soothing gargle for a sore throat.

To combat bad breath on sleep-deprived mornings, use the tea (see above) as a mouthwash. It also helps to combat gum problems. Chew on a few seeds when you don't have time to brush your teeth.

For gritty or sore eyes from lack of sleep, use an infusion as a herbal eyewash. Fennel has been considered as a cure-all for eye problems, especially conjunctivis, since ancient times.

Revive a tired-looking complexion with a deep-heat cleansing treatment using fennel leaves (see page 96).

LOOKING AHEAD Instead of using a commercial 'gripewater', ask your health visitor about giving fennel tea to your baby. Draw 1 tsp of cooled fennel tea (see above) into a sterilised pipette and drop doses on to your baby's tongue after a feed.

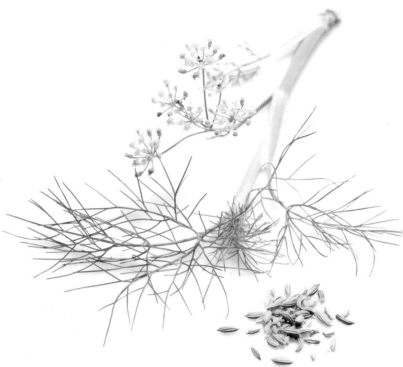

To lessen teething pain in older babies, rub the tea directly on to the gums with your finger.

OFF-THE-SHELF REMEDIES

❋ Fennel toothpaste suits sensitive gums; Green People Fennel Toothpaste is certified organic by the Soil Association. Try not to rinse or spit after the final brush, to make the most of the herb's antiseptic properties.

❋ Liquorice-flavoured aniseed tea has a natural sweetness that is tempting even if you feel bloated. Salus Haus teas, made in Bavaria, are certified organic and combine fennel with anise and caraway seeds, both valued to ease flatulence and bloating.

❋ To benefit from fennel's carminative effects when you or your partner lack time to make fennel tea (sree above), use a ready-made tincture – take 2–4 ml up to three times a day.

❋ For a morning pick-me-up, look out for fennel-flavoured honey, and use to sweeten other herbal teas, or dilute with boiling water and a squeeze of lemon juice.

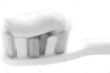

✳ For a tasty aid to digestion after a meal, try sugar-coated fennel seeds, available in Indian stores.

✳ Italian savoury *farallucci* biscuits baked with fennel seeds are good to snack on during feeds.

Cleansing steam

Fennel has a cleansing and toning action on the skin. There are claims that this plant also has powers of longevity and youthfulness – it's an old English wrinkle treatment. The lavender is added for its cleansing and calming powers, and to lift exhaustion. An extra-deep cleanse with steam feels good after the exertion of labour, and can soften a clenched jaw and furrowed brow.

1 tbsp fresh fennel leaves
1 tsp fennel seeds
2 tbsp dried lavender flowers

Fill a large bowl with boiling water and drop the fennel leaves and seeds and lavender flowers into the water, stirring them around. Place your face about 45 cm above the bowl and cover your head with a towel, trapping the steam inside. Remain under the towel for up to 5 minutes,

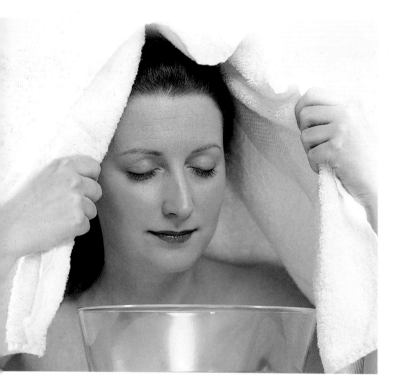

breathing deeply through your nose (keep your mouth closed if you can).

Pat your face dry with a soft towel and lie down if you feel light-headed. This is a good moment to apply a facemask, if you have time. Otherwise, simply moisturise – a few drops of rosehip oil will feel soothing and nourish the skin.

Tummy-calming tea

The lemon balm in this tea relaxes stomach cramps while the fennel seeds help to expel wind and build a good supply of milk. Having a good rest while you drink the tea will also help to increase your milk supply.

20 g dried lemon balm leaves
10 g fennel seeds
500 ml boiling water

Place the herbs and seeds in a pot or jug with a lid and pour over the boiling water. Replace the lid and allow to steep for 10 minutes. Strain into a cup and drink up to 5 cups a day.

Fennel oil

It's easy to infuse fennel leaves in oil to make a mild-flavoured base for salad dressings. They impart their medicinal properties as well as a mild, sweet aniseed flavour. You will need two dry sterilised 250 ml jars and a 250 ml bottle, all with lids.

2 good handfuls of fresh fennel leaves
250 ml extra-virgin olive oil

Pick the leaves late in the day, when they are dry, and discard any that look brown, wilted or diseased. Don't wash the leaves; they need to be completely dry.

Finely chop the leaves and place in a dry, sterilised jar. Pour over enough olive oil to reach the top of the jar (to discourage the growth of mould), making sure that every part of the leafy material is covered – stir around with a knife to 'pop' any air bubbles.

Put on the lid and label and date the jar. Place in direct sunlight to macerate for at least 2 and up to 6 weeks. Shake daily.

GROW YOUR OWN

The culinary plant Florence fennel is a different variety (*F. vulgare azoricum*) but shares some of the medicinal properties, and its umbrella-shaped yellow flowers and aniseed-scented feathery foliage make it an attractive plant for a summer screen. Florence fennel likes a sunny position sheltered from wind, and may need staking as it can grow to 1.5 m or more. Dig up the bulb early in the season and roast, chop into salads or use the bulb and feathery fronds to stuff or marinade fish; it pairs especially well with oily fish, cutting through the strong flavour to whet the appetite and aid digestion. The plant is perennial and self-seeds successfully, so you may never have to plant more than one.

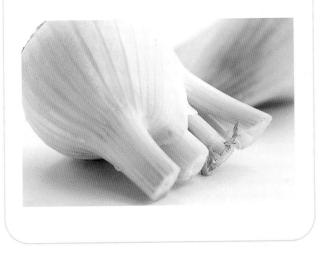

Strain the oil through a muslin-lined sieve or funnel or using a jelly bag (see page 7) into another sterilised, dry jar. Discard the leafy matter. Again put on a lid, label the bottle and store in a cool place for a week. Decant the oil into the bottle, leaving behind any watery liquid that has settled at the base of the jar. Put on the lid, label and store in a cool, dark place until ready to use.

Fennel seed mix

Munch on a pinch of this Indian mouth-freshening seed blend, or *mukhwas*, if you find that meals bring on heartburn. All the seeds have beneficial properties for the digestive system, and they are thought to be cooling to the body and mind. Sugar-coated fennel or anise seeds are traditional; if you can source them, mix in once the other ingredients have cooled.

1 tbsp fennel seeds
1 tbsp dill seeds
1 tbsp cumin seeds
1 tsp cardamoms, crushed and seeds removed
2 cloves, ground to a powder using a pestle and mortar

Heat a dry frying pan over a medium heat, until hot. Dry-fry the fennel seeds until fragrant and brown, stirring with a wooden spoon to prevent burning. Remove from the pan and set aside to cool. Repeat with the dill and cumin seeds in turn. Mix all the roasted seeds together, then stir in the tiny cardamom seeds and clove powder. Once cool, store in an airtight container. Use within two weeks.

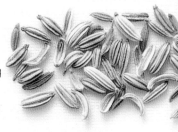
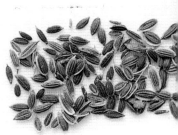
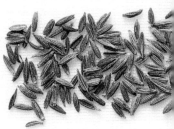
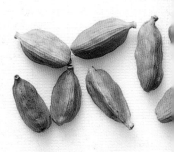
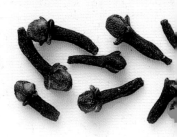

Jasmine

promoting recovery, easing depression

Jasmine is a flower of love and of the night, and in the language of flowers it means 'I attach myself to you' – what better scent to see you through the long nights of those first weeks of your baby's life.

The sweet-scented flowers and oil of this exotic climber of the Oleaceae family have a relaxing, sedating effect on the nervous system, and are valued for easing tension, treating exhaustion and lifting depression. In aromatherapy, jasmine (derived from *Jasminum officinale*) is regarded as one of the most sensual oils, which is why it is so popular in perfumery. Jasmine oil has a heady quality, and is emotionally healing, helping to restore positivity, and boost confidence and assertiveness, which can dissolve as caring for a new baby takes precedence. The scent of jasmine builds a sense of being able to cope following childbirth and the trauma some women feel at the loss of their pre-baby freedom. It can also ease the worry and doubt that come with the demands of caring for such a precious new life.

Jasmine oil is recommended by aromatherapists for balancing hormones and relieving postnatal depression, as well as for promoting a good flow of milk and relieving feelings of heaviness in the breasts. The oil is a uterine tonic, and may be helpful in calming after-pains and cramps – it can strengthen contractions in childbirth and has analgesic properties. The oil has particular benefits when applied to the skin, and is often recommended for dry or sensitive skin, especially when those conditions are exacerbated by stress.

Jasmine tea derives from a related species (*J.sambac*) and is blended with green tea, for its floral scent. The drying tea leaves are covered in jasmine flowers overnight, when the jasmine has most fragrance and therapeutic properties, in order to best absorb those qualities. This is repeated over several nights. The resulting tea is said to clear the mind and reign in overactive senses, leading to a sense of calm clarity, useful at this intense time. It is also

CAUTION Jasmine oil is intoxicating so use only in low dilutions. Avoid synthetic jasmine oil (produced for use in perfumery); this does not have any medicinal qualities.

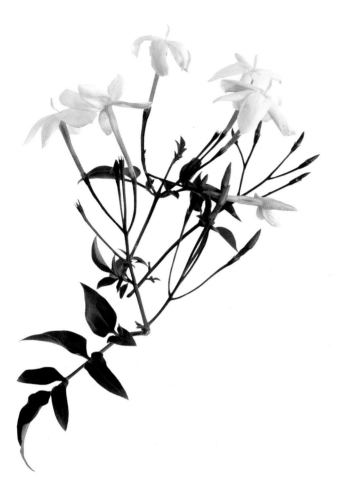

To speed healing of stretchmarks, make the massage oil blend, substituting essential oils of lavender (2 drops) and mandarin (1 drop) for the geranium, a traditional and beautifully scented stretchmark blend. Rub into affected areas after a bath or shower.

If you have a cold or cough, drink jasmine tea, reputed to cut through mucus, clear congested sinuses and support deep breathing.

To boost energy, make the most of jasmine tea's energising qualities, use loose leaves and let them brew for no longer than two minutes to keep the infusion light in taste. Remove the leaves and save to make a second brew. Some people prefer the milder taste of second or third brews.

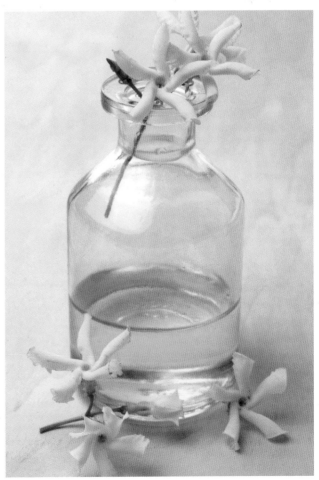

reputed to have spiritual properties, hence its role in traditional, formal tea ceremonies. Avoid jasmine teas scented with jasmine essence rather than the flowers.

PLANT TIPS

❊ *J. officinale* is the species to plant (you might find it named *J. officinale* f. *affine* or *J. grandiflorum*). This species needs a sunny, sheltered site and in less than the mildest of winters might need raising under glass. To extract the maximum scent, leave the flowers in oil overnight or simply wear them in your hair.

❊ Jasmine flowers are picked at night when they have the most intense aromatic properties and greatest quantities of indol, the deep-scented low note in this distinctive scent.

USING THE HERB

To restore confidence and the ability to cope, have a full body massage with a blend of oils including jasmine. Try the oil blend or foot balm on page 101.

To bathe sore or tired eyes, use jasmine teas; it has a long history of use as an eyebath.

To scent the hair and tame unruly locks, use the jasmine hair serum (right). In India, jasmine flowers are worn on auspicious occasions and used as offerings to honour special people.

OFF-THE-SHELF REMEDIES

❋ When choosing essential oil, look for jasmine absolute, with the botanical name *J. officinale*. The oil is very expensive because the enfleurage extraction process is so lengthy and requires a huge number of flowers to yield a tiny amount of oil. If you are looking for a cheaper option, buy 5 or 10 per cent dilutions from a reputable supplier of essential oils for therapeutic use.

❋ French jasmine oil from Grasse is especially high quality and the most likely to have been extracted in the traditional manner without solvents, using the enfleurage technique of maceration in oil.

❋ The quality of jasmine tea is determined not by the jasmine flowers, but by the quality of the green tea with which it is blended. The best are named varieties or sorted by grade, and mixes with white tea, such as white needles or silver tip (the champagne of the tea world); these are a treat. They contain more beneficial antioxidants to help your system get back to full fitness. White tea is low in tannin and caffeine, too. This tea is best drunk without milk or lemon.

❋ Seek out jasmine soaps hand-milled using the traditional cold-process method from vegetable oils such as olive, castor or coconut oil plus certified organic ingredients that preserve the skin-friendly glycerine in the product. They are likely to be free from irritating synthetic surfactants (foaming ingredients) such as SLS (sodium lauryl sulfate), and therefore kinder to delicate or damaged skin

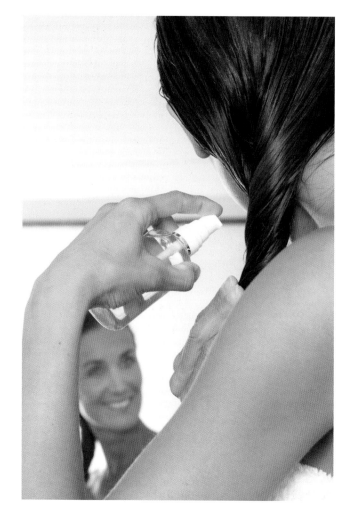

Jasmine flower hair serum

Jasmine is considered a rejuvenating hair and scalp oil throughout the East, from India to Indonesia and China, where women oil their hair before bed and roll it up with jasmine flowers. Overnight the flowers impart their medicinal properties into the oil – a method known as enfleurage. You will need a 100 ml dry, clean dark glass bottle.

1 tbsp coconut oil

2 tbsp jojoba oil

1 tbsp avocado oil

6 drops essential oil of jasmine

Pour all the oils into a bottle and drop in the essential oil. Put on the lid and shake well to combine. Label and date, then store in a cool, dark place. To use, shake the jar then pour about ¼ tsp into the palm of one hand and warm between your palms. Apply to calm frizzy locks, on dry ends to add shine or massage into the scalp once a week before shampooing as a conditioner or treatment for dandruff.

Jasmine and geranium massage oil

Essential oil of jasmine has a warming and restorative quality that feels nurturing. Geranium also works to balance the hormones and nervous system; it can help to lift depression and support female reproductive health. In Ayurvedic medicine the excess vata energy of the postnatal period (symptoms include feelings of shakiness, extreme fatigue and generally being overwhelmed with almost grief-like symptoms) is eased by warmth, stillness and routine. The latter may seem impossible right now, but a daily massage with oil at the same time most days really helps. Try to keep it up for at least 2 – but preferably 6 – weeks after the birth. This treatment is best after a warm bath.

6 tbsp (uncoloured) sesame oil
3 drops essential oil of jasmine
3 drops essential oil of geranium

Warm the sesame oil by standing the bottle in a mug of hot water. Test the temperature just before using, to check that it is not too hot. Measure 6 tbsp into a bowl and stir in the essential oils until well dispersed.

Ask your partner to give you a massage with the oil for 5–10 minutes. It is traditional to apply the oil to the head, but you might prefer to have your feet and lower legs massaged (to boost circulation), or your hands or lower back (which feels comforting).c
Tell your partner not to worry about getting the strokes right – it's more important that they feel nurturing: they should be slow and firm, flowing and repetitive, to quieten your nervous system. Keep a warm hot water bottle on your abdomen if it feels comforting.

After the massage you might like to wrap a long, wide cotton scarf around your abdomen, from hips to rib cage, as if swaddling yourself. This is used in Indonesia during the postnatal period to encourage the organs back into a pre-pregnancy position.

Jasmine and frankincense foot balm

Smother your feet in this waxy balm and then put on slipper socks – heat helps to activate the oils so their heady scent will linger all evening. Jasmine is particularly suited to very dry skin. You will need a 120 ml sterilised glass jar with a lid.

2 tbsp beeswax, grated
2 tbsp olive oil
2 tsp sweet almond oil
4 tbsp geranium hydrosol
5 drops essential oil of jasmine
5 drops essential oil of frankincense

Place the grated beeswax in a heatproof bowl. Suspend over a pan of simmering water, add the olive and almond oils and stir until all the wax has dissolved into the oil. Remove the bowl from the heat, pour the contents into another, cool, bowl, and whisk as it cools and solidifies. Add the geranium hydrosol little by little, whisking all the time until well blended – this can take some time, and you may need to put the bowl back over the pan to reheat the mixture a little. Stir in the essential oils and spoon into the jar. Once it has cooled, put on the lid and label. This will keep for up to three months.

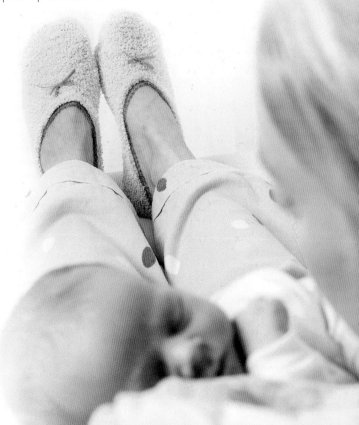

Honey

healing wounds, rebuilding stamina

A little propolis would be applied to the stump of the umbilical cord in earlier centuries to prevent infection. Bees use it to sterilise the cradles in which their babies are raised.

Honey was recognised as a cure-all for wound-healing as far back as around 50 BCE, by the Greek physician and herbalist Dioscorides. Honey is considered such an effective healer that it is still employed in hospitals across the world to dress wounds that are difficult to keep free from infection or slow to heal. Some case studies have shown it to be more effective than topical antibiotics and to offer better pain relief, less inflammation, fewer scars and quicker healing than conventional treatment. Honey's viscosity forms a protective barrier that prevents cross-infection and keeps tissue moist, providing optimum conditions for repair. It also contains enzymes that produce nature's disinfectant, hydrogen peroxide, stimulating cells to repair damage and destroying bacteria. Honey's natural acidity kills germs, and it reduces inflammation while boosting the immune system. Constituent lactobacilli may also contribute therapeutic properties.

The colour of honey
This depends on the plants on which the bees feed and the method of production.

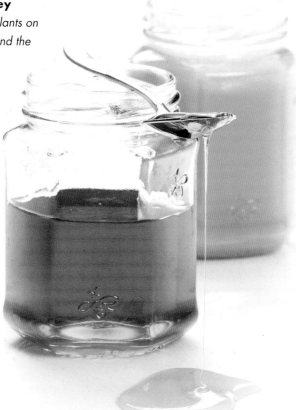

Athletes take honey to beat fatigue, aid endurance and speed recuperation – all necessary in the postnatal weeks – because of the way it helps the body store glycogen and regulate blood-sugar levels. While boosting energy, honey also soothes the digestion and sedates the nervous system.

Other products from the hive share these amazing medicinal properties. Beeswax is anti-inflammatory and pain-relieving. Bee pollen, the 'mother's milk' fed to baby bees, is a favoured stamina food of athletes, packed with vitamins, minerals and more protein by weight than any other food. It has anti-inflammatory, antibacterial and antifungal properties, too.

Red-brown propolis, the sticky varnish used by bees to glaze the hive and fix up holes, has been nicknamed 'bee penicillin' for its antibiotic, wound-healing, anti-inflammatory and immune-stimulating action.

Royal jelly, food of the infant queen, also has antibiotic properties, and works on her DNA to transform an ordinary baby bee into a queen 40 times larger than usual and so fertile she can lay six eggs a minute through her fertile years.

To reap the many therapeutic benefits of honey, eat or drink 2–3 tbsp of the 'raw' variety (see page 105) daily. When using to sweeten hot drinks, wait until the liquid has cooled a little to preserve the therapeutic properties.

USING THE HERB

For rehydration after childbirth, drink hot water sweetened with honey. One trial found honey to be more effective for this purpose than over-the-counter rehydration remedies.

For rebuilding strength and energy, add plenty of chopped dates and 1–2 tbsp honey to porridge. Bee pollen acts as an energy tonic; dissolve 1 grain beneath your tongue and build up over a few weeks to 1 tbsp daily.

To ease constipation if fear and pain are causing you to hold everything in, eat honey on toast, in yogurt and stirred into tea. For an whole-body tonic, take a 500 mg capsule of royal jelly daily or, even better, $\frac{1}{16}$ tsp of the fresh or frozen variety, mixed with honey or whizzed into a smoothie to disguise the bitter taste. Over several weeks build up to $\frac{1}{4}$ tsp (or equivalent) daily.

CAUTION Some people are sensitive to pollen – start by taking one grain. If it doesn't trigger symptoms such as itchy skin or a runny nose, increase the dose. Start with low doses of propolis and royal jelly, too. Avoid both if you are taking blood-thinning drugs, such as warfarin.

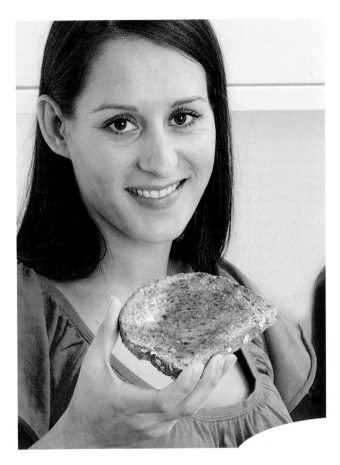

To treat inflamed skin or areas of bruising around the perineum, gently rub in propolis cream.

If your complexion is in need of revitalising, try the face mask on page 105.

For more restorative sleep, stir 2 tsp honey into milk before bed. Honey is thought to be the best fuel for storing glycogen in the liver – this feeds the brain overnight and prevents the release of stress hormones.

To speed wound healing, make a honey dressing by smearing 'raw' honey (see box on page 105) on to a gauze bandage and wrapping around the wound. Change daily. Apply to perineal stitches each time you change a pad or liner. For cracked nipples, smear on to a breast pad but wash off before breastfeeding your baby.

To counter mid-afternoon slumps (which may strike at any time if you are sleep-deprived) eat honey rather than

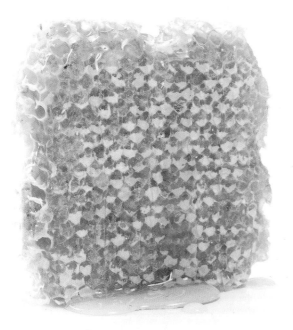

House of honey
*Available whole, halved or as a chunk,
the comb holds honey within its cells.*

a sugary snack. Studies suggest that the body tolerates honey better than sucrose (found in processed food), and that honey keeps blood-sugar levels more stable.

If stress and lack of sleep are making you forgetful, eat more honey. Research on animals has shown that replacing sucrose with honey seemed to decrease anxiety and improve memory function. Try royal jelly, too; it contains acetylcholine, lowered levels of which are associated with short-term memory loss and lack of concentration.

To treat hands made dry from nappy changing, try the softening hand salve on page 106.

For severe nappy rash apply neat raw honey. Propolis cream is good for rough or dry skin and rashes including nappy rash; also try the healing balm opposite.

LOOKING AHEAD After your child's first birthday, try offering 1 tsp of buckwheat honey before bed if a cough triggered by a respiratory infection interrupts his or her sleep. In a research study this was found to be more effective than over-the-counter cough remedies.

OFF THE SHELF REMEDIES

❋ All bee products are likely to be purest when produced in remote regions of the world far from environmental pollution. This includes the peninsula of Cornwall, New Zealand and parts of Canada. Only buy products that cite the exact source of production. However, when buying hive products to help relieve hayfever and other allergies, choose those from as close to home as possible. They're more likely to contain the pollens you react to, and are more helpful for desensitising your body than something from another continent.

❋ Beeswax is available in bars from health stores. Grate before use to thicken ointments and creams. It keeps in water, so is useful in moisturising very dry skin, such as on the feet. Use beeswax candles to give your home a honeyed scent.

❋ Bee pollen is easiest to administer in grain form – you can easily increase the dose from 1 grain upwards. To begin, let it dissolve under your tongue; when you start taking larger amounts, stir into muesli, yogurt and smoothies. Keep pollen in the refrigerator or freezer to prevent spoiling. When buying pollen look for raw, unprocessed grains or granules – air-dried and frozen types retain most therapeutic properties. Capsules and tablets are less reliable.

❋ Royal jelly is available as tablets, but is best bought fresh (look in the chiller cabinet in your local health-food store). When buying fresh online, ask for delivery in thermal packaging.

❋ Propolis is easiest to use in tincture form for colds and flu; alcohol-based products contain more propolis than water-based ones. For general well-being, chew or swallow 1–2 chunks of raw propolis daily. Both tincture and chunks can stain the teeth, so it is best to squirt down the throat or swallow whole. Capsules of propolis powder (1000 mg) are also available – take 2–3 daily for general well-being. To treat a sore throat, look for propolis essence spray, specially blended for sore throats. One squirt into the throat can also ease sore sinuses, teeth and gums.

Hive healing balm

This combines all the healing products of the hive in one supercream. Perfect as a spot-treatment cream and for relieving eczema, it also soothes nappy rash, thanks to its antibacterial and antiseptic ingredients. The beeswax base locks in moisture and gives the skin a protective coating; the orange blossom water lends an uplifting fragrance. You will need a 500 ml sterilised glass jar with a lid.

225 ml orange blossom hydrosol
25 ml propolis tincture (made with water, not alcohol)
1 tbsp raw honey
1 tsp royal jelly powder
1 tbsp bee pollen granules
50 g beeswax, grated
250 ml grapeseed oil

Combine the orange blossom water and propolis tincture in a jug and whisk in the honey, royal jelly powder and pollen granules until dissolved. Place the grated beeswax in a heatproof bowl. Suspend over a pan of simmering water, add the grapeseed oil and stir until all the wax has dissolved into the oil. Remove the bowl from the heat, pour the contents into another, cool, bowl, and whisk as it cools and solidifies. Add the water mixture to the warm oils little by little, whisking all the time until well blended – this can take some time, and you may need to put the bowl back over the pan to reheat the mixture a little. When everything is well amalgamated, spoon into the jar. Once it has cooled, put on the lid and label, then store in a cool, dark place. This will keep for up to three months.

Versatile beeswax
Available in blocks, beeswax can be grated for use in ointments or polishes and for candle making.

TYPES OF HONEY

Look for unpasteurised or 'raw' honey, which has not been heat-treated – pasteurisation and processing techniques like ultra- or super-filtration and heating destroy the healing properties. This means, unfortunately, that most supermarket honeys – even organic ones – are not useful medicinally. Distinguish raw honey by the specks of grainy pollen on its surface or cloudy haze of propolis. Jars containing lots of 'debris' have greater medicinal powers; favour those that look cloudy or marbled. Honeys sterilised using gamma-radiation retain their active ingredients.

Darker honeys – lavender, heather, rosemary, thyme – have most bioflavonoids and minerals, and greater antibacterial effects. Manuka honey, made from the flowers of *Leptospermum scoparium*, is famed for its unusually high antibacterial activity. The Unique Manuka Factor on the label rates the honey's antibacterial activity – factor 12 has been used in medical trials as a treatment for infected wounds.

Royal jelly face mask

This revitalising and nourishing mask helps to calm and soothe irritated or stressed skin. Royal jelly is ideal for a washed-out complexion. It contains vitamin B5, vital for destressing, and gelatin to fuel collagen production.

½ tsp fresh royal jelly
1 tbsp raw honey, local if possible
1 tbsp olive oil

Mix the royal jelly into the honey. The jelly will smell sour, but the honey should disguise this. Stir in the olive oil. Apply as a mask to the face or hands, avoiding the eye and mouth areas (though eating this mask can only do you good!) and relax for 10 minutes. Splash off with warm water.

Hand-softening salve

There's a lot of hand washing involved in looking after an infant. This protective lotion relies on honey's ability to attract and hold in water. Sandalwood oil is good for dehydrated skin and relieves associated itching. You will need a 120 ml sterilised glass jar with a lid.

1 tbsp honey
2 tbsp beeswax, grated
1 tbsp wheatgerm oil
4 tbsp rosewater or rose hydrosol
1 tsp apple cider vinegar
6 drops essential oil of sandalwood

Place the honey and grated beeswax in a heatproof bowl. Suspend over a pan of simmering water, add the wheatgerm oil and stir until all the wax has dissolved into the oil. Remove the bowl from the heat, pour the contents into another, cool, bowl, and whisk as it cools and solidifies. Add the water and cider vinegar to the oil mixture little by little, whisking all the time until well blended – this can take some time, and you may need to put the bowl back over the pan to heat the mixture a little. When everything is well amalgamated, stir in the essential oil and spoon into the jar. Once it has cooled, put on the lid, label and date. Store in a cool, dark place. This will keep for up to three months.

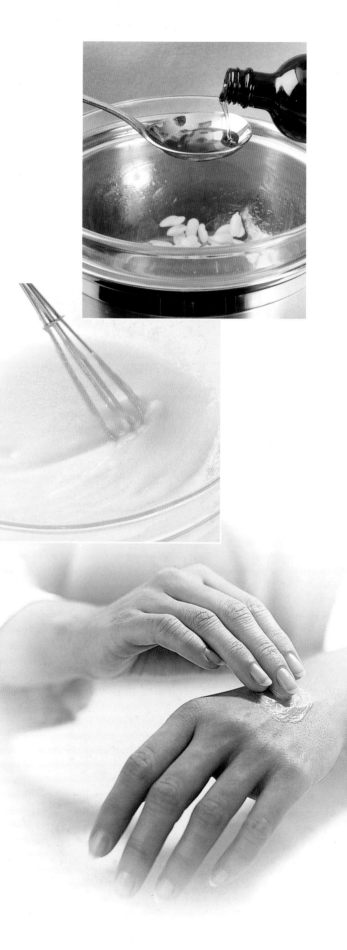

Part 7

HERBS FOR YOU AND YOUR NEW BABY

Herbs for shock and excitement, to bolster immunity,
keep you well nourished and help you cope with nausea

Catnip

soothing colic, calming

The Mohegan and Cherokee peoples of North America are thought to have been the first to relieve colic with an infusion of catnip leaves, and they also valued this herb's sedative properties.

CAUTION If picking catnip from the wild, take an identification guide with you: it's not safe to give other members of the mint family to children under five. High doses can cause excessive drowsiness and irritability.

Given its name and reputation, the perennial herb *Nepeta cataria* is probably best known for the euphoria it engenders in cats – when the leaves are bruised, a scent said to resemble cat hormones is released. As far back as 1633, English herbalist John Gerard described how cats 'rub themselves upon it, and wallow and tumble into it, and also feed upon the branches very greedily'. The heart-shaped leaves and purple-spotted white flowers may stimulate euphoria in new parents because of its calming effect on colicky babies. This member of the mint family is recommended by herbalists for soothing colic and calming a fractious infant. Colic affects about one in five babies, and is more common in first babies and boys. Symptoms include determined crying, leg-kicking and wind, and continue for more than three hours at the same time daily for at least three exhausting days a week. It can begin as early as two weeks but usually passes by the fourth month.

Catnip is rather sweet-tasting and minty, which makes it pleasant for children, and its mildly calming effects result from its carminative and anti-cramping properties. It expels painful wind in the digestive tract and relieves spasmy pain. Catnip is a gentle sedative too, encouraging body and mind to rest, and its mild nervine properties may help to calm the hyperactivity, restless legs and nervous crying in colicky babies. It may even encourage sleep! In studies on chicks, giving catnip in low to moderate doses caused them to fall asleep. But, given higher doses they became more wakeful...

Catnip is often recommended for treating colds, flu and fever. Herbalists consider it a respiratory support herb and decongestant, and it stimulates sweating to bring down a fever. A constituent of its essential oil, beta-nepetalactone, which gives the plant its distinctive scent, is valued for its insect-repellent powers.

USING THE HERB

To calm colicky crying, make catnip tea by pouring 250 ml of hot (not boiling) water over 3 freshly picked leaves. It's important not to boil this herb; instead, let it sit in hot water for 5–10 minutes. For a stronger infusion use 1 tsp of the dried herb, allowing it to steep for 5 minutes. Either drink yourself, if breastfeeding (2–3 cups daily), or, once cooled to milk temperature, give 1 tsp in a sterilised pipette with an older baby's feeds.

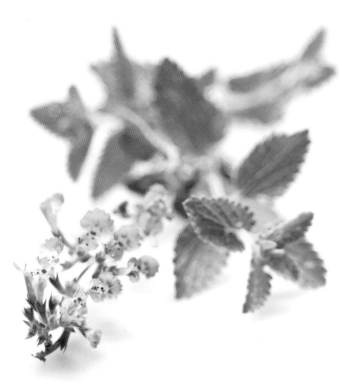

Warm baths can help soothe the crying and leg-kicking that accompany colic – add a cup of catnip tea (see above) to the water.

For calming the gastrointestinal tract and relieving wind, make a tea blend with catnip and chamomile (see page 110). This can be useful if colicky crying is giving you stress-induced digestive symptoms.

To encourage rest if you feel sleep-deprived, make a chamomile and catnip blend tea (see page 110), allow to cool slightly, then soak a flannel in the brew, squeeze out and apply as a compress to your forehead.

For tension headaches brought on by the sound of crying or interrupted sleep, sip a strong cup of catnip tea (see left), but allow it to cool first.

To ease pains or pre-menstrual symptoms exacerbated by stress or lack of sleep, when your periods return, try drinking catnip tea (see above).

To reap all the benefits of this herb, add the raw leaves to salads – it's good combined with other mints and parsley in tabbouleh and other Middle-Eastern-style salads.

At the first signs of a cold or flu, drink a hot cup of catnip tea (see left).

GROW YOUR OWN

You can find carnip growing wild on roadsides and wasteground and by streams, but it is easy to grow your own. Catnip thrives, like mint, in most sites and soils, but prefers sun, and doesn't need the same level of moisture as most mints. Pick fresh leaves before the plant flowers (from mid to late summer) for a mild flavour; after flowering the scent is more pungent. To dry the plant, harvest the whole flowering top in high summer and hang upside down until the leaves are dried; drying leaves are said to repel rodents.

Cut the stems back hard after flowering and the plant will produce a fresh set of leaves in late summer. The plant self-sows extraordinarily well, so it might be advisable to plant into the ground in pots. Thanks to its insect-repellent properties, the plant is said to be good for companion planting around cabbages, squash and cucumbers.

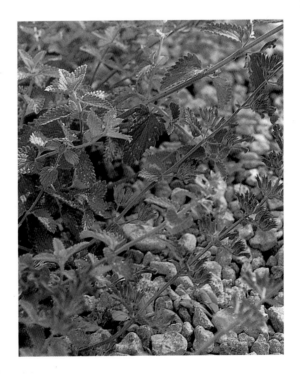

To ease respiratory symptoms, hayfever and sore throats, use a strong infusion as a steam inhalation. To treat these symptoms in infants, add ½ cup to bathwater.

For cold and flu symptoms and fevers, use the catnip cordial recipe (right).

If you are trying to avoid petcare treatments based on pesticides, try washing the coats of your pets with a strong infusion of catnip to deter fleas.

For an instant insect and ant repellent, rub the skin with a leaf. In studies, catnip has been found to be one of the most effective natural mosquito repellents.

Speed the healing of minor cuts and grazes and soothe insect bites by swabbing the area with cooled catnip tea. Its tannins aid tissue repair.

OFF-THE-SHELF REMEDIES

✳ Symptoms of colic can respond well to massage with tincture of catnip mixed into olive oil (see opposite).
✳ When hayfever triggers sore, gritty eyes, try to rest for 10 minutes with some used warm catnip tea bags over your eyes.
✳ For adult insomnia, look out for eyebags and sleep pillows filled with a blend of herbs including catnip. Don't give pillows to your baby.

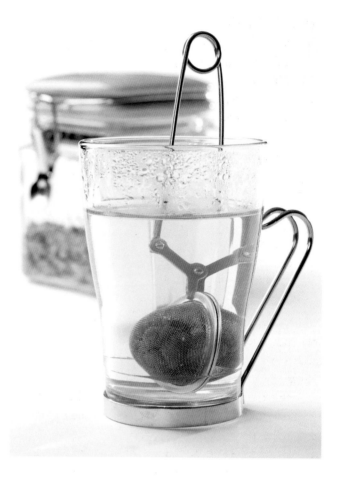

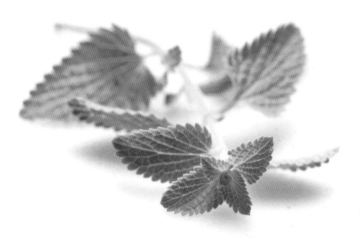

Catnip and chamomile tea

The German chamomile in this tea relaxes cramping while the anti-flatulent catnip relieves wind. Use water which has boiled but is not boiling; boiling is said to spoil the flavour of this herb. You will need an airtight container with a lid.

3 tbsp dried German chamomile (*Matricaria recutita*)
1 tbsp dried catnip
1 tsp raw honey, optional

Combine the dried herbs and store in the airtight container. To make tea, place 1 tsp of the mixture in a mug, pour over boiled water and allow to steep, covered, for 5 minutes. Sweeten with honey, if desired.

Catnip cordial

This is a favourite syrup for reducing flu symptoms, mucous and a fever, and is said to gain in effect from the combination with elderflower (*Sambucus nigra*). Elderflowers have relaxant properties and produce a slight perspiration to reduce fever while helping the nose and throat to resist infection. Lemons are added for their cold-busting properties and lemonade-like taste. You will need two 500 ml sterilised glass bottles with cork stoppers.

20 g dried or 30 g fresh catnip
500 ml boiled, not boiling, water
500 g caster sugar
juice of 1 lemon
1 unwaxed lemon, sliced
12 heads of elderflower, rinsed well

Place the catnip in a teapot or jug and pour over the boiled water. Put on the lid and allow to infuse for 10 minutes.

Place the sugar in a large pan. Pour over the strained catnip infusion and gently heat, stirring, until the sugar is dissolved. Stir in the lemon juice and slices and the elderflower heads. Cover and leave to cool for 24 hours.

Strain through a muslin-lined sieve into the sterilised bottles. Seal with the cork stopper, label and store in a cool, dark place. To use, give ¼–½ tsp 2–3 times daily, with feeds. Dilute half and half with boiled water if you prefer.

Catnip massage blend

Massage can be an effective way to calm both a colicky baby and a stressed parent. It helps if your baby is used to massage, so do try the same strokes when he or she is not stressed, for example after a morning bath. Some small babies dislike being undressed; if so, do the strokes over clothing at first without using oil. For preference, use organic olive oil on baby skin, and wait until 30 minutes have passed after a feed.

1 tbsp extra-virgin olive oil
3–5 drops tincture of catnip

Place the oil in a small bowl and stir in the catnip drops very well. Place a little oil between your palms and rub them together to warm it.

With the flat of your hands, stroke up one side of your baby's abdomen to the navel, with one hand following the other. Repeat on the other side.

Place your first two fingers beside your baby's navel and press gently. Then slide around a few centimetres in a clockwise direction and press again, Repeat, sliding and pressing around the navel, circling outwards until you reach the right hip.

Finish by making large circles, up from the right hip to the ribcage, across the chest, then down to the left hip and across. Repeat several times.

If your baby finds strokes on the tummy uncomfortable, turn your baby over, tummy to your thighs, and stroke around the lower back instead, in a clockwise direction.

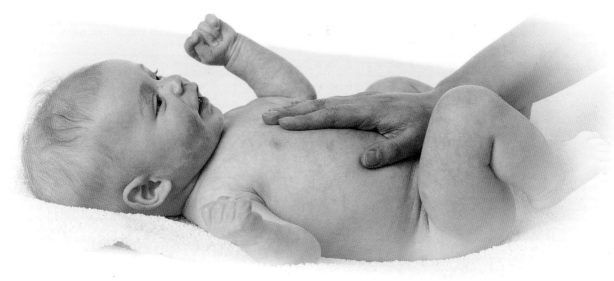

Aloe vera

softening and regenerating sore skin

The Arabic name for one type of aloe, *saber*, is said to translate as 'patience' – a useful quality at this stage of motherhood.

Fondly known as the 'first-aid plant', the succulent aloe (*Aloe barbedensis*) contains a clear jelly-like substance that can be safely applied directly to the skin – even delicate baby skin – to help heal wounds and skin conditions. This emollient gel swiftly relieves irritated skin, stimulating healthy cell regeneration in injured areas, while its bactericidal and fungicidal properties help ward off infection. Aloe gel also seems to dampen the perception of pain, boosts the immune system and has anti-inflammatory properties, hence its reputation as a 'cure-all'. For babies, the herb's ability to speed healing and kill bacteria makes it invaluable in the nappy area while, for mums, it can also ease postnatal skin problems.

Aloe vera gel is good for preserving that pregnancy glow when applied to your skin. In controlled trials, studies showed that applying the gel to the skin increased collagen – the skin's protein – by 93 per cent.

PLANT TIPS

※ An aloe vera plant can be raised in a pot on a windowsill. The exotic pendulous orange flowers are dramatic, but you will need green fingers to get it to flower!

INSTANT REMEDY

To extract the gel from the inner part of an aloe vera plant, just snap off a leaf and split it open, then press out the gel with a blunt knife. Smear directly on the skin. Alternatively, use a commercially prepared product from health-food stores or online; look for a 'pure aloe vera gel' content of 99–100 per cent on the label.

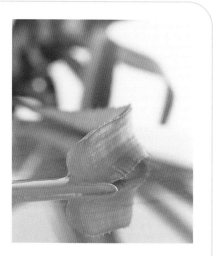

✳ Cultivate the plant indoors if you are worried about air pollution. Unlike most plants, it continues to digest carbon dioxide and give off oxygen during the hours of darknessk making it suitable for a bedroom.

USING THE HERB

To keep the nappy area clean and problem free, use the babywipe lotion and treatment gel (see page 114).

To improve hair quality, ease cradle cap and for scalp problems in general, dab some gel on to affected areas.

To treat stretchmarks and dry skin and ease pregnancy-induced varicose veins, apply the gel daily to the affected areas.

For holiday insect bites and sunburned skin, smooth the soothing gel over the skin.

To cleanse wounds, grazes or burns, use 'neat' gel, then add a protective layer of gel or a dressing soaked in gel.

OFF-THE-SHELF REMEDIES

✳ Look for gels with the word 'aloe' or its Latin name (*Aloe barbedensis*) high up the list of ingredients, and favour those containing 98 per cent or more aloe gel. The best commercial preparations are organic, cold-pressed and contain 100 per cent gel. Neal's Yard brand is good. Avoid products made from 'aloe-vera extract'. In trials, off-the-shelf gels have not proven as effective in healing damaged cells as gel squeezed fresh from a leaf.

CAUTION Avoid if you have haemorrhoids or kidney problems, and do not use during pregnancy. Occasionally aloe vera can cause itching of the skin; if this occurs, discontinue use. Do not take or apply 'bitter aloes', aloe juice or latex (from a different part of the plant) which is used medicinally as a strong laxative and purgative.

TREATING NAPPY RASH

Aloe vera gel not only is a remarkable skin-healer, it leaves a protective layer on the skin and reduces the risk of infection. This is great for babies who suffer with nappy rash. If you're using a commercially prepared gel, choose one that does not contain alcohol (which stings). Use three to five times daily.

If your baby suffers from soreness or redness or reacts to conventional nappy rash creams, at every nappy change, wash with plain water only or natural babywipe lotion (see page 114). Pat dry or dry with cool air from a hairdryer, then apply just enough of the gel to cover the clean, dry skin. Don't rub in, but allow to air dry before putting on a clean cloth nappy.

If your baby's bottom is really raw, cleanse with aloe vera gel then soak a cloth nappy liner in gel and place next to the skin.

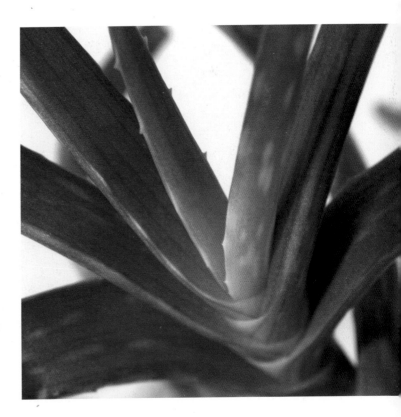

❋ Aloe vera toothpaste is recommended for bleeding gums.
❋ Aloe extract cream (0.5 per cent) should be applied three times a day to promote the healing of cold sores and psoriasis.

Natural babywipe lotion

This gentle cleanser suits sensitive bottoms, and is soothing on the skin. You will need a clean reusable glass bottle with a spray-pump top. Keep refrigerated and make up a new batch every three days.

2 organic chamomile teabags
1 tbsp hemp oil
1 tbsp aloe vera gel

Put the teabags in a teapot and pour over boiling water. Allow to infuse and cool for 15 minutes.

Transfer 30 ml of the lukewarm tea to a jug and add the hemp oil and aloe vera gel, then whisk well to combine all the ingredients.

Pour the mixture into the bottle, screw on the top and shake well to combine all the ingredients again. Use immediately or allow to cool completely before storing in the refrigerator.

At nappy changes, shake the bottle well, then spray a little of the lotion on to unbleached cottonwool or a cloth wipe and use as much as you need to clean your baby's bottom.

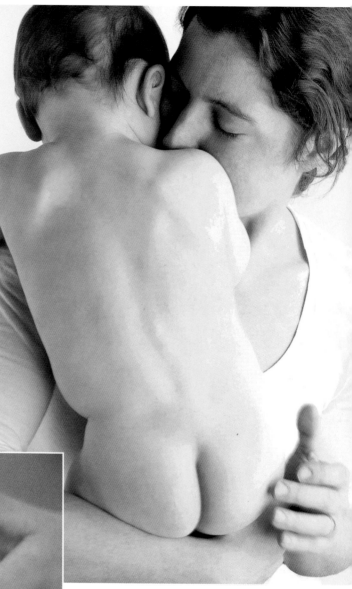

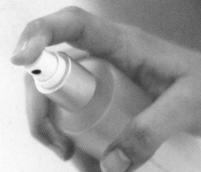

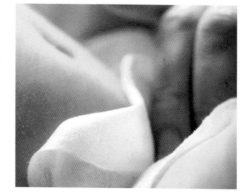

Olive

softening, boosting well-being

The olive is one of the oldest cultivated trees and its leaves have been used since ancient Greek times for wound cleaning and healing.

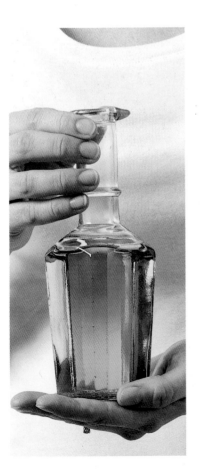

The emollient oil from the fruit of the evergreen olive tree *Olea europaea* is traditionally recommended not only as a method of delivering herbs (it forms the base of ointments and liniments and 'carries' essential oils) but as a softening treatment for very dry or inflamed skin, from stretchmarks to nappy rash. The constituent unsaturated fatty acid squaline, which also occurs in human skin, is believed to boost suppleness and counter environmental damage. The huge numbers of antioxidants in the oil – largely flavonoids, but also vitamin E – are valued in skincare preparations. Its soothing and softening properties also protect the digestive system and make the oil valuable as a gentle laxative, while its antimicrobial action can ease gastrointestinal problems.

The consumption of olive oil is most often associated with a Mediterranean diet, and the benefits this has for cardiovascular health. To benefit your own health, use it as your everyday fat of choice – about 3 tablespoons will benefit the cardiovascular system. Nutritionally, olive oil is praised for its omega-9 monounsaturated fatty acids (primarily oleic acid, but it is the phenolic compounds in the oil that produce its famed anti-inflammatory, antioxidant and anticoagulant effects, and help blood vessels to relax and dilate. The phenolic compounds also seem to benefit bone health and have an antimicrobial action on food-borne pathogens. The stinging sensation at the back of the throat in peppery extra-virgin olive oil indicates the presence of oleocanthal, the pain-relieving and anti-inflammatory powers of which are similar to those of ibuprofen.

The astringent leaves of the tree are also used medicinally – they contain higher concentrations of many of the active ingredients than the fruit, particularly phenols – and researchers are looking into using leaf-extract to treat bacterial and fungal infections, lower blood pressure, regulate blood-sugar levels and as a general tonic for improved well-being.

CAUTION Avoid olive oil if you know you are allergic to other plants of the Oleaceae family such as privet and lilac.

USING THE HERB

For post-pregnancy heartburn or 'hyperacidity', add olive oil to food; its emollient properties soothe the digestive tract and it seems to reduce gastric secretions.

As a gentle laxative, olive oil is useful; just use as your cooking oil of choice, and add the dressing opposite to your salads.

To moisturise stretchmarks – and dry skin generally – rub olive oil into the affected areas once or twice a day; this is most effective after a bath or shower. Wait for a while before dressing to allow the skin time to absorb the oil.

As a hair treatment, use 2 tbsp warmed olive oil to massage the scalp (add 3 drops of essential oil of rosemary if you have dandruff). Or just coat very dry or colour-treated hair or split ends with a little oil. Wrap your hair in an old warmed towel and relax for 20 minutes if you can. Then shampoo twice. You probably won't need conditioner.

For cradle cap, rub olive oil into your baby's scalp once or twice a day, or use the cradle-cap oil opposite.

OFF-THE-SHELF REMEDIES

※ To maximise the medicinal action, choose extra-virgin olive oil. These are cold-pressed – no heat or chemical solvents are used – preserving the therapeutic properties. Heating yields more oil, but of poorer quality. Oil in dark glass bottles or opaque tins is likely to contain greater amounts of beneficial phenolic compounds.

※ If you would like to try olive-leaf extract – as a mild diuretic or for cystitis – the recommended dose is 5 ml diluted in water, three times a day.

※ The Bach Flower Remedy Olive is recommended for the total exhaustion that follows intense periods of activity. When life with a small baby brings you to the point when you feel you can no longer cope, add 2 drops to a glass of water and sip as necessary, until you feel more energised.

※ Olive oil soap is very good for baby skin. Look for bars milled in Mediterranean regions.

GROW YOUR OWN

Olive trees prefer a Mediterranean climate and free-draining soil, but since they thrive in dry, rocky places and drought conditions, they can do well in pots, even if neglected. In cooler climates, however, trees may not produce fruit. They do better on the coast and in warm cities. You may need to bubble-wrap the container if temperatures regularly drop below freezing for long periods. Every year consider transferring the tree to a slightly larger pot or top dress it by scraping away a layer of soil and replacing with fresh compost and a layer of mulch.

Nappy rash ointment

This ointment combines the skin-softening properties of the olive tree with chickweed, to harness this herb's fat-soluble ingredients which are effective for soothing very inflamed skin. You will need an ovenproof bowl with a lid and two 250 ml sterilised glass jars with lids.

25 g beeswax, grated
250 ml extra-virgin olive oil
50 g dried chickweed

Place the grated beeswax in an ovenproof bowl. Suspend over a pan of simmering water, add the olive oil and stir until all the wax has dissolved into the oil. Remove the bowl from the heat, stir in the dried chickweed, making sure it is well covered, and put on the lid.

Put in a low oven for three hours, then strain through a muslin-lined sieve into a bowl, pressing with the back of a spoon to extract as much oil as possible (or use a jelly bag in a jug, see page 7). Decant into the jars and, once cooled, put on the lids. Label and date and store in a cool, dark place. Use liberally after cleaning the nappy area.

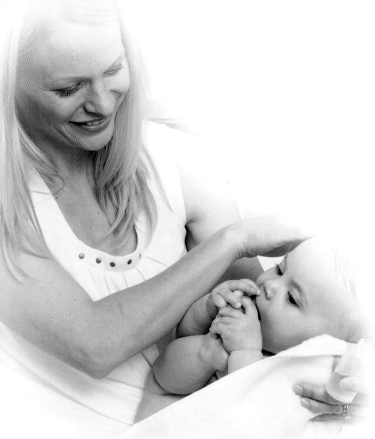

go rancid). Squeeze the contents of a vitamin E capsule into each bottle. Lid, label and date. For extra strength, repeat the process using this infused oil with a new batch of catnip.

To use, warm a little of the oil between your palms and gently rub into your baby's scalp. Leave on for 15 minutes, then shampoo. Never pick at patches of cradle cap.

Salad dressing

Oiling your body from the inside is a great idea if your skin is feeling dry. Use this recipe to dress green salads and to cut through oily fish dishes (you should be eating oily fish such as mackerel, salmon, trout and herring twice a week if you are breastfeeding).

MAKES ENOUGH FOR 1–2 SALADS

1 tbsp balsamic vinegar
6 tbsp extra-virgin olive oil
juice of ½ lemon
pinch of herbes de Provence
1 tsp Dijon mustard
1 tsp raw honey (see 105)
sea salt and freshly ground black pepper, to taste

Spoon the vinegar and olive oil into a glass jar with a lid and squeeze in the lemon juice. Add the dried herbs and shake well until everything is combined and viscous. Stir in the mustard and honey, whisking well with a fork to combine. Season with salt and pepper, then taste and add more honey or lemon juice as necessary. Use immediately, or refrigerate for up to a week.

Cradle cap oil

Herbalist Nicholas Culpeper wrote of catnip that 'the head washed with a decoction taketh away scabs, scurf, etc'. This scalp oil combines those properties with the soothing and antimicrobial qualities of olive oil. You will need a 500 ml glass jar with a lid and two 250ml sterilised glass bottles, with lids.

250 g fresh catnip (unwashed but dirt removed)
500 ml extra-virgin olive oil
2 vitamin E capsules

Chop the catnip as finely as you can (or pulse in a blender until roughly chopped). Place in the glass jar, then pour over enough olive oil to cover all the green matter and reach to the top of the jar. Use a knife to 'pop' any air bubbles. Put on the lid and store in a warm, dark place for at least 2 and up to 8 weeks, shaking daily. The longer it stands, the more concentrated the active ingredients.

Strain the oil into a bowl through a muslin-lined sieve, pressing with the back of a spoon to extract as much oil as possible (or use a jelly bag in a jug, see page 7). Return the oil to the jar and leave overnight. Next day decant into the bottles, leaving any green particles of sediment in the base of the jar (they will cause the oil to

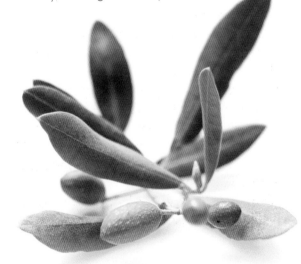

Thyme

disinfecting, cough suppressing

The 17th-century herbalist Nicholas Culpeper declared thyme a 'notable strengthener of the lungs' and said there was no 'better remedy growing' for whooping cough in children.

The mauve flowers and aromatic foliage of the evergreen shrub garden thyme (*Thymus vulgaris*) are among the most potent antiseptics and antimicrobials of the herb world, and have a long history of use in remedies for the upper respiratory tract, including bronchitis and tonsillitis. Thyme has a taste children find pleasant. As an expectorant, it encourages excess mucus from the bronchial tubes, while ingredients in the volatile oil, including thymol and methyl chavicol, plus flavonoids help to relieve muscle spasms. Since it is a 'bitter' herb with carminative properties, thyme can be helpful for digestive discomfort, too, from indigestion and wind to gastritis. It can be used to expel worms in older children (though you probably don't want to think about that yet).

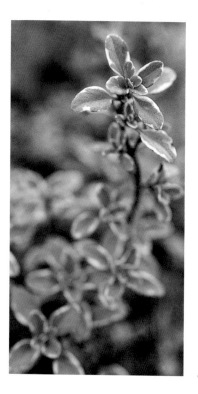

Thyme gains its powerful antimicrobial properties from rich amounts of volatile oil, and in studies, extract of thyme has been active against listeria and salmonella as well as effectively inhibiting *Clostridium botulinum*, *E. coli* and *Candida albicans*.

The herb also acts as an overall tonic for fatigue, fortifying all the body's systems with its natural warming action – have a cup of stimulating thyme tea when you feel in need of a pick-me-up. It is particularly effective for complete exhaustion and loss of concentration, and when spirits are low – the ancient Greeks regarded this herb as an emblem of activity and vigour. There is some evidence that thyme also has anti-ageing properties – it's certainly a potent antioxidant. It has

been a favourite in perfumery and beautycare since ancient Greek times – the name in fact derives from the Greek *thumos*, meaning 'fragrance'.

USING THE HERB

Clean nappies and work surfaces with antibacterial thyme using the recipe on page 120.

To relieve catarrh or a chesty cough, make an infusion using 1 heaped tsp of fresh thyme leaves to 250 ml boiling water. Allow to steep for 5–10 minutes. Give 1 tsp three times a day after the age of six months. From age one, 3 tsp three times a day is recommended. The adult dose is 3 tbsp three times daily. This may also relieve asthma symptoms.

For night-time congestion, stir 1 drop of essential oil of thyme into 1 tsp of grapeseed oil and drop into a bowl of warm water. Placed near the bed but out of reach, so your child can inhale the fumes.

For a sore throat, chew on a sprig of fresh thyme or gargle with an infusion for its antiseptic properties.

In hayfever season or during bouts of asthma, start the day with a cup of thyme tea.

Ease diarrhoea by drinking a cup of thyme tea after a meal; its astringency is thought to be helpful.

To gain from all thyme's positive qualities, use it in slow-cooked dishes, such as casseroles and stews, bakes and roasts – add a bouquet garni (see page 121). The flavour marries well with tomato and seafood. Add to marinades for barbecuing (using the lemon-scented variety for fish dishes) and press into bread dough before baking.

For adult fungal infections such as athlete's foot and ringworm, mix 2 drops of essential oil of thyme into 1 tsp of grapeseed oil and apply to the affected area. For thrush, apply 2 ml of the tincture two to three times a day.

Clean wounds with an infusion of thyme – the antimicrobial properties and astringency are useful aids to healing. Make use of these antimicrobial properties to disinfect nappies (see page 120).

To promote hair growth and deter dandruff, massage an infusion into the scalp before washing your hair. It also makes a great toner.

Harness the insecticidal properties of thyme by filling small cotton bags with the herb. Place them between wool and silk clothing in drawers and wardrobes to deter moths.

Bathe insect bites and stings with a strong brew of thyme tea (see left) to relieve itching.

To boost energy and help to keep you awake, drink an infusion of thyme, or pour it into a bath.

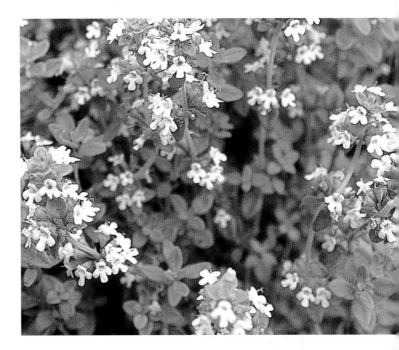

To lift a low mood, pour 1 tbsp grapeseed oil into a small bowl and stir in 5 drops of essential oil of thyme and 3 drops of essential oil of rose. Pour into a bath and swish well to disperse before stepping in.

OFF-THE-SHELF REMEDIES

* Honey made from thyme flowers has a wonderfully aromatic flavour.
* Look for olives marinated with thyme leaves. Thyme also adds its preservative powers to meats such as sausages and patés.
* Substitute thyme teabags for regular tea or coffee to promote a positive attitude in the morning. Salus House organic teabags use medicinally graded herbs.

CAUTION The essential oil can be an irritant when used topically. Avoid both the oil and large doses of the herb during pregnancy and if you have high blood pressure. Thyme reduces milk supply, so use sparingly while breastfeeding.

GROW YOUR OWN

Thyme is an essential herb for the kitchen garden. It has a lovely creeping habit that makes it suitable for ground cover, but it grows well in pots and windowboxes, or even directly in a wall – simply push young plants between stones. In a garden this is a perfect plant for attracting bees and other beneficial wildlife. Thyme plants prefer light, dry conditions and will tolerate less than rich soils and drought, but they do require full sun. Harvest the flowering tops and leaves from mid-summer, when the plant begins to flower. Hang the stems upside down in a cool, dry place until dried. Alternatively, freeze freshly harvested summer sprigs to use in winter when the plant stops growing. Both freezing and drying retain the aroma and flavour of the fresh herb.

Prune well to stop the plants becoming 'leggy', but don't cut back into dead wood – the plant will not revive.

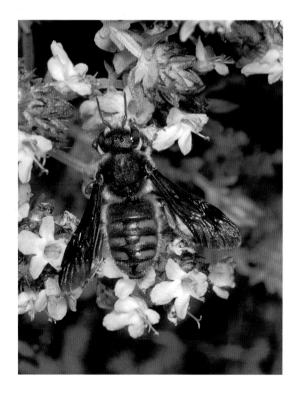

Thyme nappy disinfectant

Call on the powerful antimicrobial properties of thyme to sanitise cloth nappies if you are using washables. The herb has been used since Roman times to disinfect and up until World War II the oil was employed in hospitals for its antibacterial and antiseptic powers. Lemon also has an antibacterial action. You will need a bucket with a lid.

4 tbsp bicarbonate of soda
4 drops essential oil of lemon
4 drops essential oil of thyme

Half-fill the bucket with water, then stir in the bicarbonate of soda, until dissolved. Add the essential oils, then use as an overnight soak for used nappies before washing as usual.

If you prefer to use as a disinfecting wipe for surfaces, add the same amount of essential oils to 1 tbsp witch hazel in a 100 ml plastic bottle with a pump-action spray, then top up with distilled water. Shake well before use.

Thyme cough syrup

The thyme in this recipe acts as an expectorant, but the syrup is soothing in itself for a sore or tickly throat, especially at night. You will need two 500 ml sterilised glass bottles with cork stoppers.

30 g fresh thyme
500 ml boiling water
500 g unrefined sugar

Place the thyme in a teapot or jug with a lid and pour over the water. Put on the lid and leave to infuse for 15 minutes.

Strain the infusion into a saucepan, squeezing the herb to release as many of its active ingredients as possible. Place the pan over a medium heat and add the sugar, stirring until it has dissolved. Keep heating until the mixture develops a syrupy consistency. Remove from the heat and allow to cool.

Decant the syrup into the sterilised bottles, seal with the corks, label with the name and date and store in a cool, dark place. For adults take 4 tsp 3 times a day. For infants over six months old, give ½ tsp three times a day; for infants over a year give 1 ½ tsp three times a day.

Thyme toner

In beautycare preparations, thyme is valued for its astringency (due to the constituent tannins) as well as its tonic nature. This toner also counters infection and irritation.

40 g fresh thyme sprigs
500 ml water
juice of ½ lemon

Place the sprigs of thyme in a saucepan with the water. Bring to the boil, then reduce the heat and simmer, uncovered, for 10 minutes. Remove from the heat and allow to infuse for 5 minutes.

Strain into a jug, discarding the woody matter. Put on a lid, allow to cool, then stir in the lemon juice and store in the refrigerator for up to 48 hours. Use as you would a toner, after cleansing the skin, or apply direct to pimples and rashes using a cottonwool ball.

Bouquet garni

Throw this bundle of fresh herbs into slow-cooked dishes, such as soups, stews, casseroles and stocks, to impart a pungent taste of the Mediterranean and real depth of flavour. You will need a piece of unwaxed string.

3 large sprigs thyme
3 bay leaves
2 parsley stalks
1 stalk celery, leafy top only

Wash the herbs, then tie them together with the string and throw into the pot. Hook out before you serve the dish.

As an alternative, experiment with different taste combinations: try adding sage or tarragon for chicken dishes, lemon thyme for pork, rosemary for lamb and fennel for fish.

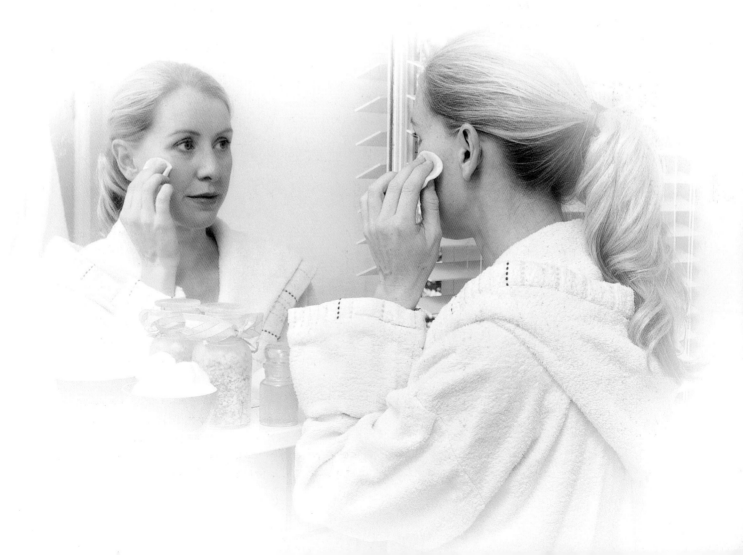

Lime flower

reducing irritability, gently sedating

In Poland, the linden tree, or *lipa*, is considered so relaxing that simply to sit in its shade soothes the soul, and the tree is considered a favourite of the blessed mother, Mary.

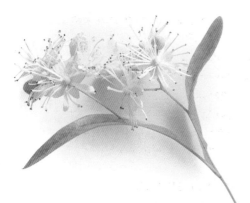

CAUTION Avoid if you have heart problems. There have been no studies to prove the safety of this herb while breastfeeding.

The pale yellow flowers of the deciduous linden or lime tree (Tiliaceae family) have such a deep and lingering fragrance that they can fill an entire neighbourhood when in bloom and bees love them. Herbalists value the flowers for calming irritable or over-excited infants and relaxing stressed or panicky parents. The flowers are harvested from a number of species of trees in the family, including the small-leaved *Tilia cordata* and large-leaved *T. platyphyllos*. *T. vulgaris* or *europaea* is a hybrid of these parent trees.

The sedative properties of lime flowers, taken as an infusion, can bring speedier sleep and a calmer mind to rest-deprived parents. The flowers are antispasmodic too, so are used to calm stress-related digestive complaints in babies, particularly colic and cramp. The blood-thinning flavonoids in the herb improve blood circulation and relax the arteries, and the flowers are also valued for their ability to shift catarrh and mucus. Both these actions can help to ease headaches: in France, a *tilleul* infusion is taken for this purpose. Lime flowers are used by herbalists to speed recovery from illness in general, but since the constituent flavonoids and p-coumaric acid promote perspiration, they are particularly useful for treating fevers. The flowers can also ease coughs and throat irritation.

The emollient quality of lime flowers makes them suitable for skincare preparations, specifically for calming sensitive or itchy skin, and their tannins are astringent.

PLANT TIPS

* The flowers of the small-leaved lime *T. cordata* can be harvested when in full bloom in high summer. It's easiest, however, to make remedies from ready picked dried flowers.

* In Germany and Poland it's traditional to plant a tree near the home for protection and to bring happiness and luck (but not too near since it grows very tall); the heart-shaped leaves make this a tree particularly associated with blessings for women.

USING THE HERB

For nervous headaches drink 1–2 cups daily of an infusion made with 1 tsp dried lime flowers to 250 ml boiling water. Allow to steep for 10 minutes before straining.

To relieve stress and nervous tension take a lime flower bath (see right) or infusions (see left).

For infant eczema and to encourage sleep, add a couple of dried lime flowers to the water when running a bedtime bath – tie them in muslin and keep safely away from inquisitive fingers. A lime-flower toy (see page 124) hung near the cot may also help your baby to sleep.

To reduce a fever, drink an infusion (see left) as hot as you can bear, to encourage perspiration.

If a stuffy nose stops you from sleeping, clear the passages by adding 4 drops of the essential oil to a bowl of hot water or a vaporiser. Alternatively, use the steam treatment on the right.

To combat puffy eyes, soak two cottonwool pads in a lime flower infusion (see left) and rest for 10 minutes with the herbal pads on your eyelids.

To reap the many benefits of this herb, try the refreshing young leaves in sandwiches.

OFF-THE-SHELF REMEDIES

❉ Look for single-blend teas from the species *T. cordata* and *T. platyphyllos*, which have the best taste.
❉ Lime flower may be found combined with other calming herbs, such as chamomile, in commercial blends.
❉ Use the tincture for (adult) insomnia, taking ½–1 tsp in water before bed.
❉ Honey from lime (or linden) flowers has a greenish tinge and is delicious, but can be tricky to track down. Poland and Lithuania (where it is known as *lipez*) are good sources. Look also for Polish candles formed from beeswax made from pollen from the aromatic blossom.
❉ Natural baby bath products may be formulated with lime flower – on the ingredients list look for lime or linden flower or blossom and varieties of *Tilia*.
❉ Burt's Bees combines lime flower with aloe for cooling and moisturising parched skin in its After Sun Soother.

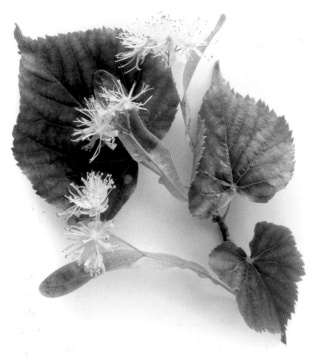

Lime-flower steam treatment

This suits sensitive skin and relieves headaches caused by blocked sinuses and nasal catarrh. You will need a warm room for this treatment – a bathroom is ideal.

20 g dried lime flowers
1 litre just-boiled water

Place the dried flowers in a large jug with a lid, pour over the water, put on the lid and leave to infuse for 15 minutes.

   Strain the infusion into a large bowl, place your face about 45 cm above the bowl and cover your head with a towel, trapping the steam inside. Close your eyes and inhale the steam, through your nose if possible, for 5–10 minutes. Relax in the warm room for a further 15 minutes to allow any catarrh to shift through your airways.

Sleep-inducing lime-flower bath

Harnessing the plant's sedative and muscle-relaxant properties, a warm bath with lime flowers is a well-known cure-all for insomnia,

30 g dried lime flowers
2 litres just-boiled water

Place the dried flowers in a large jug with a lid and pour over the water. Put on the lid and leave to infuse for 15 minutes. Strain into a warm bath just before stepping in. Let your baby lie on the floor in the bathroom to inhale the lime flower infused steam.

Elderflower and lime flower flu relief tea

This herb combination helps to push colds and flu through the system more speedily. The lemon balm combines beautifully with the slightly spicy flavour of the lime flower. Omit the lemon balm if breastfeeding; it may reduce your milk supply.

15 g dried lime flowers
10 g dried elderflowers
5 g dried or 10 g fresh lemon balm, optional
500 ml boiling water
honey, to sweeten, optional

Place all the herbs in a warmed teapot or jug with a lid and pour over the water. Put on the lid and infuse for 10 minutes. Strain into a cup and sweeten with honey to taste. Drink one cup daily.

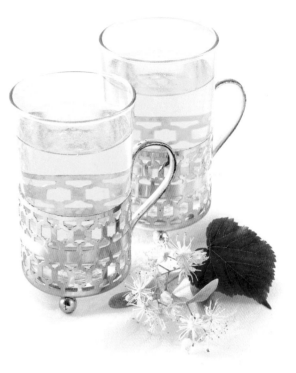

Lime-flower scented toy

The scent of lime flowers can calm a fractious baby and induce sleep. It's easy to make a simple toy to hang in the cot or tuck in a pram.

fabric remnants, including some suitable for lining
50 g dried herbs such as lime flowers, lemon balm, or catnip, or a combination of your choice
ribbons and/or other trimmings

Draw a simple shape or follow a pre-existing template (you might find something in a magazine). Pin the shape to your doubled-over fabric and then cut it out so you have a front and a back. Right sides together, stitch the two shapes together, leaving a gap of a couple of centimetres. Turn right sides out and press flat. Repeat with lining fabric, and use this to line your animal. Fill with the lime flowers or other herbs. Stitch the small gap closed. Decorate if you wish, then hang on to the bars of the cot with a short length of ribbon, away from inquisitive fingers.

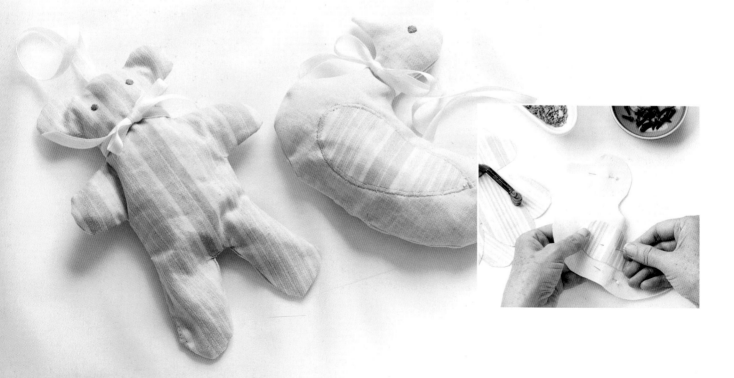

RESOURCES

ONLINE INFORMATION

National Center for Complementary and Alternative Medicine (NCCAM)
http://nccam.nih.gov
Sponsors research studies into complementary and alternative therapies, including herbalism, and offers 'Herbs at a Glance' fact sheets detailing what the science says about specific herbs and botanicals. Offers 'search a database' of possible herb–medication interactions.

Medline Plus
http://www.nlm.nih.gov/medlineplus/druginfo/herb_All.html
Features profiles of medicinal herbs, with reports on their use, efficacy, usual dosage and drug interactions, offered in conjunction with the US National Library of Medicine and the National Institutes of Health (NIH). Rates herbs according to whether they are likely to be safe in pregnancy and while breastfeeding.

Dietary Supplements Labels Database
http://dietarysupplements.nlm.nih.gov/dietary/
Provides a database of research studies about herbs and plant ingredients, including those used in selected brands of supplements, with information on the action of plants on the body and any adverse effects.

American Pregnancy Association
http://www.americanpregnancy.org/pregnancyhealth/naturalherbsvitamins.html
The association's remit is to promote pregnancy wellness, assessing herbs and supplements considered safe for use during pregnancy.

Plants for a Future
http://www.pfaf.org/user/default.aspx
A resource and database of edible and medicinally useful plants. Check out the week's top-rated edible botanicals and medicinal plants.

The Herb Society
http://www.herbsociety.org.uk/
Set up more than 80 years ago to increase understanding and appreciation of the health applications of herbs, the society offers information on growing as well as medicinal and cosmetic uses.

American Botanical Council
http://cms.herbalgram.org/healthyingredients/index.html
Independent research and education organisation dedicated to providing reliable information on medicinal plants for consumers and practitioners. Profiles plants used in dietary supplements and natural cosmetics on its Healthy Ingredients page.

RHS Plant Finder
http://apps.rhs.org.uk/rhsplantfinder/
Run by the Royal Horticultural Society, this is the first place to go for information about sourcing and growing plants, organised by botanical name.

The Wild Flower Society
www.thewildflowersociety.com
Includes a useful code of conduct for foragers.

Susun Weed
http://www.susunweed.com/
The doyenne of using herbs for fertility, in pregnancy and for healing during the postnatal period. Note particularly her article 'Herbal Allies for Pregnant Women'.

SUPPLIERS OF HERBS AND BOTANICALS

G. Baldwin & Co
http://www.baldwins.co.uk
Long-established London herbalist with mail order service. The website includes an A–Z of health notes and prescribing guides, plus a newsfeed.

Jekka's Herb Farm
www.jekkasherbfarm.com
Specialises in organic plants and seeds – over 650 varieties to buy online.

Bach Flower Centre
www.bachcentre.com
For the original Dr Bach flower remedies and information on their use in pregnancy.

Quinessence Aromatherapy
http://www.quinessence.com/
Offering the finest organic oils sourced from ecologically grown plants, this is the choice of many professionals.

Dr Hauschka Med
http://www.dr.hauschka-med.de/english/about-drhauschka-med/
http://www.dr.hauschka-med.de/english/quality/plant-library/
For the BDIH-certified (the German Association of Industries and Trading Firms) natural cosmetics developed with dermatologists, aestheticians, dentists and independent testing laboratories to ensure substances are active and have an holistic effect on the body. Many of the medicinal herbs are sourced from the biodynamic herb gardens developed along anthroposophical principles. The online plant library contains fascinating profiles of herbs used in the products.

Weleda
http://www.weleda.co.uk/
Established in 1921, this company creates herbal and homeopathic remedies based on anthroposophical principles and using only natural ingredients, grown biodynamically where possible. Their baby products are excellent.

Inlight Organic Skincare
http://www.inlight-online.co.uk
Offers the Dr Spiezia range of products, which are organic as standard and informed by homeopathic principles, made on a farm in Cornwall by potentising oils then steeping herbs in them.

Neal's Yard Remedies
http://www.nealsyardremedies.com/
Supplier of herbs and remedies (and the equipment for making them), plus award-winning natural and organic cosmetics, for more than 30 years.

Index

Entries in **bold** denote main herb profiles

ACKNOWLEDGEMENTS

Special thanks to my husband and daughters for giving me time to write and being willing subjects for experimentation. Thanks to lovely editor Anne Yelland, Chrissie Lloyd for her designs and, as always, to Amy Carroll for her inspiration.

PICTURE CREDITS

Photolibrary.com
pp2–3; p22 top and bottom; p29; p36; p37; p39; p42; p44; p51; p52; p53; p55; p57; p62; p78; p81; p82; p86 bottom; p87; p93; p99 top and bottom; p100; p104; p113; p114 top, middle and bottom; p120.

Getty Images
p21.